May ...
"Beau...

Patricia

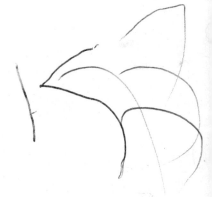

Shake, Rattle & a Cinnamon Roll

by
Patricia A. Schauder

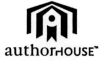
authorHOUSE™

1663 LIBERTY DRIVE, SUITE 200
BLOOMINGTON, INDIANA 47403
(800) 839-8640
WWW.AUTHORHOUSE.COM

First published by AuthorHouse 11/18/05

ISBN: 1-4208-7876-X (sc)

Library of Congress Control Number: 2005908054

Printed in the United States of America
Bloomington, Indiana

This book is printed on acid-free paper.

I would like to thank my mom for never giving up on me. Mr.Jerry Campbell, who taught me more than textbooks, did? I want to thank my three siblings, who have encouraged me to persevere through out my life, Al Gall, the Westgate Village Shopping Center, all the smiles that passed my way, Sariah, who helped me finish my first book, and Connie Webster who kept me on the straight and narrow. Teresa Grossi, who never stopped believing in my abilities and kept running with me to catch my dreams. Paula Coleman and Karen Gryzca who saw me as I truly am. Names have been changed to preserve some relationships.

"Friendship"

And in the distance you might hear a deaf man sing

as church bells ring throughout winter's wind

Why?

Ask me again in ten thousand years

and I shall answer once more, It's not a game!

It's not money, fortune and fame!

It's a tear in the darkest of night!

A small child consumed by fright!

Must we fear the answers to why?

Accept the fact that in order to gain

we must surely forfeit a friend or lover!

but yet we still crave the warmth of another.

In order for a seed to bloom

it must surely feel the bittersweet rain.

Before one triumph she'll be consumed by pain!

Did you ever see a lame man fly

or a diamond sailing towards the bright blue sky?

Ponder the enchanting force encircling you and me!

One may never actually know the reason to why?

Reach out for a rose yet beware of its thorns

as time rushes on and someone else is born!

Can you view the bitter chill

of winter as it appears with a sharp cry!

Mortal man will never answer all the questions of how and why

If by chance we venture once more

deep within the core of each other

don't fear what might not be there!

Accept the fact that many will run

while only a few really care!

Touch me with the beauty of your words!

Hold me with a passionate smile

Be my friend for a very short while.

Until that moment when my dreams come true

and I thank the Lord for knowing you!

I once was but now I am! This morning I basked in the salty mid-summer heat, musing over the happenings of this past spring and summer. What is this strange, powerful force affecting every filament of my being? Was it the coming of age? The reality of womanhood? The discovery of morality?

Am I going to take control of my existence, or be swept up in the tide allowing myself to be battered on the shore, pulled out to the sea, dashed up against the jagged rocks of life or set hopelessly afloat?

Oh yes, my intellect has all the answers, the education, and the experience of a "together" person. I am the poet, the lover of each day, the unique woman of my street, always giving, deriving pleasure from all that I did for others. Suddenly, without warning, all this is not enough. I gazed deep within myself and came face-to-face with a void, an insatiable hunger for more. More books! More romance! More love! More hugs! More gentleness! More time! More attention! More beauty! More understanding! My emotional self had no answers.

Had it all began with the passionate touch of a man-child who viewed himself to be a great gigolo? Maybe it was a magnificent obsession of an illusive lover from my past. Could it have been Micheal, whose lips were so soft and caring? He vanished like the clouds soon after a warm spring rain. Was it the mere vision of Jim, the brief entanglement of paradise until death blows her kiss onto his lips? All I know now is that I must recapture that mystical power which held my senses until I begged for more!

God granted my existence! Satan had his hand at placing daggers in my vessel, this clay pot that feels, touches, and desires only to be accepted by something just beyond my reach. This invisible transformation is screaming to be held yet people only hear what they want and disregard the rest.

Table of Contents

Preface

"Cerebral Palsy: paralysis caused by brain damage prior to or during delivery, and marked by a lack of muscular coordination, spasms, and difficulties in speech," so a medical dictionary explains. People may be afflicted by various degrees of Cerebral Palsy. Some walk and just slightly shake. Others, like me, are severe and need practically every physical activity done for them. This way of life does not affect the mind, yet people tend to assume that since my body doesn't function the way theirs performs, I don't have any faculties. I learned, way back in my childhood, that the act of assuming makes a total jackass out of you and me. We all have flaws in some way or another. In this society not many will take credit for a flawed being, like some dent in a Ford, so she's put in a junkyard! If I am to be the woman, God created, then it's going to take time for me to get up and rolling!

Can you ever imagine fighting your own spasms when trying to accomplish an activity of daily living or physically fighting with yourself in order to put your clothes in the washer? Pressing the buttons on a calculator feeling like you're sitting in an earthquake. This is how I felt all my life. The most painful of all was sitting in the back of a church looking at others hugging, laughing and embracing one another. I was not included because others perceived me as "Untouchable," I felt contagious, similar to what Christ might have felt all through his entire journey on this earth. You may finally realize how difficult my physical disability is! How limiting society makes life for the individual that happens to have a different lifestyle.

I have a chance to go out and get those things, which I only imagined, that have walked right by me, and out the door. I merely saw life and wanted to live it. Any being with motivation has a certain pull that tears at their soul until each vision breaks into reality. I am still finding ways around this bubbling system that attempts to rule my soul. The barricades built, by intellectual idiots, forming laws by which the limited shall abide. How, you might ask. I feel nonessential, and fearful that I have committed a mortal sin, and am punished for something that was not my fault! We only have one set of rules that we must obey.

Society creates its own version of these basic commandments, that enables the rich to become wealthier, and the poor to die a slow, torturous death! Their jurisdictions build stumbling blocks between us, and the ability to convert our dreams into realities! Where did we go wrong? Each one on earth builds their own walls to protect themselves, out of fear, anger and hatred. These walls are the answers to each of our circumstances. I have been behind a societal wall for the majority of my life. My blame is the lack of knowledge, I was never aware of my rights. I, finally, learned this information that made me who I am today. A woman free to live her life, the way she chooses to! Society's attribute is the lack of money and time. This excuse seems simplistic to resolve. I am determined to take responsibility for my shortcomings, shattered my walls through my personal struggle. What's societies problem?

As we grow, we imitate those around us. We dream of making love to affluent men, and experiencing life like John Boy. We mature with the thought that everybody cares, and no one tells tall tales, leaving you with broken impressions of what they want for you. Where did I go wrong? What question was one too many? I only saw life and wanted to live it. And now I ponder over my whole situation, for a lengthy period of space, and during that meditation I discover that I am not doing what I want and when I want to do it. I'm too busy doing what others tell me to do. What I want is what God grants me!

What am I asking? I merely want to experience life on my own terms. I hate taking valuable time away from another whole individual. For example, when I lived with fifty other residents, and we only had one staff for every ten residents. When I needed a staff member, all the other nine residents were neglected. I felt like I was on a time clock all the time. This is not how I felt God wanted me leading my eighty some years on this earth. I must find a way around this bubbling system that attempts to rule the life that God granted me. At one time, my staff was required to document my meals, medication, toileting, and even who contacts me over the telephone, as well as the reason they contacted me. I had no privacy so my provider of services can receive funding to assist me in my daily life.

This was where my dreams enter like the winter snow creeps through the autumn wind.

A well-known lecturer once taught me a lot about the ability to form, and nurture, relationships. He stated once, "If you have one best friend who you can turn to, consider yourself fortunate! Someone you could talk to about anything, or to give you a hug when you think no one cares, blessed are you! You might just require a new viewpoint on the situation that you're almost sure you won't come through. Society is programming us to do everything ourselves, never revealing to others that we are weak!"

It's strange how some people can cope with more pressures than you can count, and others will break down if only faced with one or two? If you drown your troubles with alcohol, cigarettes or working twenty-three hours a day, you aren't confronting your situation head on. I am as guilty as the next. I recall getting letters from my Godmother Wilma. Wilma was a good Christian woman, yet each letter told of some tragedy that would strain any soul! There are times when I ponder why God would grant anyone such as Wilma so many bad happenings.

It took me years to figure out that God doesn't send these stressful experiences, Satan creates these problems in hopes that we will fall away from His love. Satan is the biggest jerk alive! He preys on the weak to make us think that God isn't as loving as His Word states. Think of it. Christ was as human as you or me. He laughed as well as cried bitterly over each being on the face of the earth! Over 2000 years ago, this baby didn't have a sterile, germ-free, hospital to be born in. He slept in a manger right next to cows and sheep enveloped by the aroma of a barn. He had great joys as well as being brutally beaten until he bled to death for us!

We tend to neglect the fact that Christ came to this earth as a mortal man. He was tempted in all ways, besides having to experience the whole gambit of emotions that we deal with on a daily basis. This life is a massive chess game where God and Satan are the competitors with each person being a king, queen, rock, bishop, knight or pawn. God is all-powerful, yet we tend to think He's only around at the great times, when you give birth or finally get the job you wanted. Wrong! God is with us even in the darkest corners, when we think Satan has us in checkmate. There are times when I wonder where God is. It's these times when He's carrying me! My friend, we cannot conquer all our trials-of-life on our own!

Second Corinthians 12:10 states, "Therefore I am well content with weaknesses, with insults, with distresses, with persecutions, with difficulties, for Christ's sake, for when I am weak, then I am strong."

I will never live up to this world's expectations. Now a days, you must have large breasts and look like a Barbie doll in order to be considered someone! You must wear skintight jeans and have at least two pounds of make-up on before you might get a second glance from anyone of the opposite sex! I remember Karen Carpenter, who was a popular singer of the '1970s'. Each time I saw her, I cried inside because she was so thin. I wonder if she was ever happy? After her death, in 1979, I learned that she had a disease called Anorexia Nervosa. I ponder if she developed this to gain attention from the public eye? I hate this world, with all its conditional loves. Christ accepts me the way I am!

Many people, who have never actually come in contact with physically challenged individuals, somehow get the impression that they are sick! At least once a week, a man by the name of Jr. would tell me that he's praying for my healing. This always puzzled me. In order to be healed, you must be sick first! God could perform a miracle by taking my Cerebral Palsy away tomorrow yet there would still be something wrong with me! No being on this earth is without some form of limitation. We are created in His image, yet because of the fall of man in the Garden of Eden, everyone is disabled in some way or another. The idea is still very discouraging. Why am I consistently looking for acceptance in my life?

Chapter 1

The Awakening

But they that wait upon the LORD shall renew their strength; they shall mount up with wings as eagles; they shall run, and not be weary; and they shall walk, and not faint.

Isaiah 40:31

It all began, one cold and snowy November night. My dad and mom were in their small fifth floor apartment when mom went into to labor for the sixth time that day. This was when I am making my grand entrance into this world.

"I think it's time to go to the hospital, dear." mom gave dad a big smile.

Lynn, my older sister, couldn't understand why mom would not stop crying. My dad, was doing his best to comfort mom while, he attempted to keep Lynn entertained. Lynn was only eighteen months and was a true tomboy.

Dad called Wilma, to baby-sit Lynn, so he could take mom to the hospital. Wilma R. would soon become my Godmother. She was expecting this call. Wilma lived around the corner from our first house in Woodville, Ohio.

One of my first memories is when she used to baby-sit me. Wilma would have a box of buttons that I played with while I laid on the floor. When I started crawling around reaching for the buttons, my head got caught under her sofa. I thought I was never going to get free. Wilma came to the rescue, as she always had, that time by lifting the end of the couch to release my head.

Mom and dad would play cards every Saturday night, with a few other parents, so Wilma would use a large chest of drawers as beds for all the children. After all, it would be hard to fall when I was in a drawer. Mom's car rolled over once and she broke her kneecap. Wilma took care of me while Mom recovered. To this day, Wilma is a beautiful human being, who I admire as an individual for everything she has been through.

Dr. Wolf, who planned to deliver me, was attending an important annual event, a fundraiser for the newly built intensive care unit. He had special interests in funding for the hospital, primarily his department, and a special interest in the hostess Helen Denardo. Dr. Wolf hesitated to leave the party thinking he had plenty of time and he had consumed one too many margaritas. His priorities as a physician were blurred and his focus was not on delivering babies, but on Helen and how radiant she looked that evening.

She was the first woman to catch Dr. Wolf's eye, since his second divorce. He was the most eligible bachelor in town, being handsome with a tall stature, dark black hair, strong facial features with a distinct dimple on his left cheek, and beautiful blue eyes. The doctor was known around town for his Casanova personality and infidelities. Helen was his objective for the evening. He had been eyeing Helen for months. He wanted her that evening, and had every intention of playing doctor in the bedroom. Shortly after his deviant thought ended, Helen was approaching him and they quietly walked upstairs trying to go unnoticed by their colleges. As soon as they were out of sight they embraced and kissed passionately.

Meanwhile, downstairs the phone rang, and was answered by the butler. The butler searched the home looking for Dr. Wolf. In a final attempt the butler looked upstairs, opening a closed door, which revealed Dr. Wolf and Helen in a compromising position. Everyone involved was embarrassed; the butler for opening the door, Helen for her inappropriate behavior and Dr. Wolf for neglecting his patients. The butler proceeded to inform Dr. Wolf that he was needed immediately at the hospital. Dr. Wolf looked at Helen as he hurriedly fastened his pants. He would merely claim that it was an act of social justice, an innocent way of showing a fascinating hostess that her party would be the talk of the town for quite some time. He turned to the butler and asked if he could go warm his corvette up for him? He would be right there. When they were alone again, Dr. Wolf reached for Helen and whispered that he had been madly in love with her, even if she was married to the chief of staff of the Intensive Care Unit of the hospital.

My mom was screaming when Dr. Wolf finally opened the delivery room doors. She was dilated to ten centimeters and I was crowning. Dr. Wolf was told that Mom was in labor and dilated to ten centimeters. He informed the nurse that they had some time in view of Mom's first pregnancy, with Lynn, when she was in labor for forty-eight hours. No one in town would ever tell Dr. Wolf, that he had consumed too much to.

"How is she doing?" Dr. Wolf asked franticly.

The head nurse looked panic stricken and said, "This baby should have been out hours ago!"

As Dr. Wolf pulled my tiny head out, his hands were trembling. I came out screaming, which was a good sign. Dr. Wolf looked at mom "It's a girl," he said matter-of-factly.

Mom watched the nurses rush her daughter to a table where they cleaned me up and wrapped me tightly in a pink blanket. A nurse brought the pink bundle over to mom. With tears in her eyes took me into her arms and happily said, "Isn't she beautiful?" Mom asked one of the nurses softly "Could someone dim the lights, it's too bright in here." As the lights dimmed I closed my eyes and fell into a deep slumber.

Before Dr. Wolf left the room he looked back from the doorway and asked Mom "What are you going to name her?"

Mom replied, "Her name is Patricia Ann, after my mother."

As Dr. Wolf left dad walked into the room. He walked briskly towards mom asking, "Honey, are you okay?"

Mom just smiled saying; "We have a beautiful baby girl!"

Dad bent down and kissed mom's lips. As Dad turned towards the door to thank Dr. Wolf, he realized that he was gone.

Dr. Wolf walked down the hall as fast as possible. His heart was racing as he told himself, "This can never happen again. I know there's something wrong. This is going to ruin my career! I will never admit it was my fault." He threw the locker room doors open pounding his fists on the walls. All Dr. Wolf could think about was his reputation, yet Helen still hadn't left his mind.

Dad and mom took me home from the hospital two days later. Every thing seemed normal at first, but by the time I was three months old I cried repeatedly and was unable to hold my head up. Concerned for me, my mom made an appointment to see Dr. Wolf.

For the first three months Dr. Wolf hid the truth about me. At my first visit, Dr. Wolf told dad and mom that my progression was normal. He knew it was time to tell my parents the truth about me. They had grown suspicious and threatened to change pediatricians.

Dr. Wolf arrived at his office and checked his schedule, as he always did before his morning cup of coffee. His smile turned to dismay when he realized his first appointment of the day was the Schauders. He decided to avoid them as long as possible by taking other patients first.

Finally, dad got up and went to the receptionist window and said, "We have been waiting for an hour and a half! Our appointment was scheduled for 9:00 a.m."

The receptionist explained, "Dr. Wolf is very busy and will be with you as soon as possible."

Dr. Wolf came to the door of the reception area and said hesitantly "Paul and Julie you can come back now. Sorry about your wait."

My parents entered his office and sat down with concerned looks on both their faces. Dr. Wolf sat down across from them clinching his hands and leaning forward on his desk. "The reason your appointment was delayed is because I needed to speak to my colleagues. We have come to the conclusion that Patricia Ann would be better off in an institution."

Mom, shocked by this response, asked the doctor, "What are you talking about? What is wrong with her?" When I couldn't hold my head up, mom began to worry. She kept me on the floor much of the time so I couldn't fall anywhere.

"Patricia Ann, we believe, has Cerebral Palsy. This means she won't amount to anything and will basically be a vegetable." Dr. Wolf explained.

Mom started to cry. Dad, trying to comfort her, put his arm around her. She threw his arm off her shoulder by standing up abruptly with me in her arms. "Who do you think you are telling me that my child should be institutionalized?" yelled mom. "How long have you known?" Mom looked down at me. "Patricia Ann is our child, just like Lynn, only she might need special treatment. We are not putting her away. She was born with Cerebral Palsy simply because you came late!" Mom pointed her finger at Dr. Wolf, "Now, you want us to just discard her like a snagged blouse." Mom turned to Dad. "He came later than Pat needed him. She only wanted to live! Look at her! Look at what some system created. The tears shed! The responsibility passed so no one is to blame and now they expect us just to put her away and go on with our lives! " She looked at Dad. "Come on dear, we will find a real doctor! Not some psychotic maniac like him!"

Dr Wolf looked angrily at the Schauders, "Anyone you take her to is going to say the same thing. You'll be better off if you put your child away because of her diagnosis with Cerebral Palsy. She will only be a vegetable and won't amount to anything when she grows up."

In my first twenty-three years of spastic movements, being fed like a baby and no great love affairs, I found a genuine belief in God. He got me through my teenage years, while my two brothers, and one sister, escaped the nightmare of dad's alcoholic lifestyle. They join their own peer groups, which left me to deal with dad all alone. There were many times that I, too, prayed to break free from that Hades lifestyle.

First, Mr. Paul Martin Schauder was my dad. You could spot him anywhere because he never wore anything but a crew cut and dark colored socks. I should know, for I had the weekly task of sorting the family's socks each Friday. Dad was an only child, which explains why Grandma Schauder didn't admire anyone who would marry her pride and joy. Dad was a military man. After graduating from high school, he joined the U.S. Air Force when WW11 began. Dad was a top gunner on a B-17 and flew over the oil fields of North Africa and Italy, among other countries, where war materials were being manufactured. He came home and married my mom on May 26, 1951, just after he was honorably discharged in 1945. Mom was one of nine children. Mom told me once that she would come home from school, at times, to hear a newborn baby crying upstairs.

Grandma Schauder was totally against Mom marrying her only child, so she got back at her by calling me Patsy every time we visited. Grandpa Schauder was the town's Key-smith and their house was right next to a railroad track. I was sitting on Dad's knee once as a train rumbled past the house. I cried, for everything shook, as if we were in an earthquake. Grandma Schauder made the best homemade noodles with chicken gravy. She was talking over the phone when she had a massive heart attack and died in 1966. I didn't go to her funeral because I had a bad cold.

My parents were great, for they knew I was slow and required special treatment. Lynn, my eighteen-month-older sister, had a very hard time understanding why Mom took more time with me than her. This was quite understandable because she had Mom and Dad all to herself for one and a half years and then I appeared! Dad and Mom took five years, after I popped into their happy home, to have Joseph. Joseph was a fine baby with deep blue eyes and golden hair. He was walking in his seventh month and by the time John made his entrance into this household, Joseph was trying to talk. This made my family complete, two boys and two girls. He raised all four kids in a military fashion. Never reveal any inner feelings, and speak only when spoken to. I was the black sheep of this clan.

I must have made the Guinness Book of World's Records because, at the age of 22 months, I began speech therapy. Some people may think this

5

was a major mistake, because I began vocalizing my thoughts. In other words people may think I have a big mouth! I can get into trouble as easy as winking my eye.

Dad sold vacuum cleaners during this stage of my life. He read an ad in the newspaper for a job with the government up in Battle Creek. This was just the break he was looking for because my parents had found a special school that dealt with disabled children. We sold our house on Woodville Road and rented one for nine months, in Sylvania Ohio, while we searched for a house that we could buy up in Battle Creek. I looked out of our front screen door one morning when this big old house was rolling down our street. I thought to myself, "Boy that's what I call moving house!"

Joseph and John entertained themselves by playing hide-and-seek in some gigantic boxes Dad kept in the garage for moving purposes. I recall Mom dressing them up as two little gangsters for Halloween one year. Mom could easily keep the two of them busy by having them paint our sidewalk with water. This worked very well until they learned about evaporation.

In 1960, my parents heard about an experimental surgery dealing with restricting spasms by opening the skull and killing cells that cause spasticity. They shaved my head twice because the doctors had to go into each side of my brain. The doctors first did the right side. I remember having to stay awake, during each operation, so that I could wiggle my fingers when they needed me to. Mom bought me a wig to wear in between the two processes that were six months apart.

Chapter 2

My Early Adult Years

1962-1968

"And not only this, but we also exult in our tribulations. Knowing that tribulation brings about perseverance, and perseverance proven character; and proven character, hope; and hope does not disappoint, because the love of God has been poured out within our hearts through the Holy Spirit who was given to us. For while we were still helpless, at the right time Christ died for the ungodly,"

Romans 5:3

It was November 22, 1963 when John F. Kennedy was in a motorcade, turning down Houston Street in Dallas, as a gunman shot him in the neck. A second shot got in his head. I was in third grade and remember seeing the news reports on our library's TV. I was startled and surprised. John F. Kennedy was rushed to Parkland Memorial Hospital where doctors tried to save him but failed. He was buried on November 25th at Arlington National Cemetery. It was J.F.K. JR's third birthday. Dad raised all four of us in a military fashion, never showing any feelings or expressing any sign of weakness. On that Monday, they televised the funeral and I saw my Dad cry. I had just turned ten the day before.

I started attending Ann J. Kellogg's Elementary School, in Battle Creek Michigan, during this traumatic period of my life. I recall my wig, somehow got caught in the heater, and it came off. The kids all laughed at my baldhead. They didn't know what to think as our aide gently reset the wig on my head as if it was a top hat. In my first year of school, I passed both my first and second grades. I was extremely bright for my age!

Jerry C. was the school's speech therapist. I recall the first time I met him. My staff pushed me into his therapy room and then walked out, shutting the door behind her. I was terrified! There I was, without Mom, alone with a very handsome man. Jerry never talked down to me but treated me like any other kid. If I did all my lessons during the week, we would play two hands of poker on Friday. We played for gumdrops. Once, the principal came in the room during one of our hot hands, and it took some quick thinking on Jerry's part. He rationalized playing this game by telling the principal that he was teaching me to say my numbers. Another kid started coming to my speech class with me. Rod was his name and he was almost identical in the Cerebral Palsy that I have. In fact, we could have been fraternal twins. We had the same attitude towards life and loved taking risks! Rod's parents bought him an album entitled "Whip Cream" by Herb Albert and the Teiwana Brass for Christmas one year. Rod was so excited to bring it to our class that he neglected the appearance of the jacket. He proudly brought the album to school and showed it to Jerry. The jacket had a naked woman on the front covered with whip cream. Jerry immediately took the cover and placed masking tape over the X rated body parts. This was my first experience with nudity, and Rod didn't really care what the lady was, or wasn't, wearing. He just loved the music.

Jerry was a magnificent trumpeter and had his own band that played on weekends. "Jerry Jumping Jacks" was the name of his five-man group and they were very well known around the town of Battle Creek. We formed our own small club, which was entitled the National Association of Rat Finks. This title terrified anyone who happened to hear it, before they found out what the letters meant. The letters stood for Responsible, Active, Talented, Friendly, Interesting, Nice and Kind. Many thought we were insulting them until we explained the meaning behind each letter.

No matter how tiny these four words are; responsible, active, talented, friendly, interesting, nice and kind, taught me much about life and accepting the inner core of a person instead of taking one glance at someone and rejecting them because their skin isn't the right shade or they're slightly plumper than Miss Twiggy. At that age, it was important to have a sense of belonging! A feeling that, if you died tomorrow, there would be an empty space in this world which no one else could fill!

Yes, Jerry was my speech therapist, yet he taught me much more than mere words can say! I worked with him on various committees in Battle Creek, after I graduated from Ann J., and even saw his band perform once or twice when they did benefit concerts. Jerry surprised me once by dedicating the song "Feelings" to me. I am very fortunate to have him in my life!

My physical therapist was a little old lady by the name of Mrs. Murphy. At the age of 10, I wore braces up to my waist and walked either in parallel bars or a walker. The walker reminded me of an opened telephone booth with casters on each of the four bottom corners. This allowed me much more freedom than the bars, plus it was less frightening. I was born without any balance, but when they stood me up and securely locked my body into this contraption, I felt safe. We would walk up and down the halls of the school. Mrs. Murphy would threaten me when we passed Jerry's opened door. She wanted to buy me a pair of blinders, something like a horse wears, so I wouldn't look all around. I always had to peek in to see if he was there and, if he was, I made some sort of noise to attract his attention. I really had a 'thing' for Jerry but never actually understood the meaning of a 'thing' until I graduated from that school.

I finally got too heavy for Mrs. Murphy, as well as Mom, to handle in those hip braces. Even Miss Gwen, the other physical therapist who worked in the same room as Mrs. Murphy, agreed that I was getting to be quite a load. Mom used to call me a 'sack of potatoes'. I don't really know what to think of that nickname and so I simply smiled whenever she would call me that.

Did you ever think of someone bathing, dressing and feeding you or wiping your butt after you used the restroom? Can you imagine your hair being fashioned the way someone else likes, and not taking into consideration that it's you who will wear it all day? Well, because of my spasticity, I'm not able to do many of the daily skills, which you take for granted. This is why I started Occupational Therapy at Ann J.

Sue D. was my first therapist in this realm of my life. In my many attempts at feeding myself, I learned that it's extremely exhausting to only get five bites in my mouth. I was ready for rest period half way through my lunch! I could never develop the talent of using a spoon but I found that by jabbing my food with a fork, I controlled a bite of meat or anything that would stay on the fork. Piercing my food was one major accomplishment, yet getting it up to my mouth was quite another story! I sometimes saw bites flying through the air with the greatest of ease while I stabbed my mouth with the fork. Feeding myself is still very hazardous to my health and so I have to be fed, which can be interesting, as well as boring, at times.

9

I tried brushing my teeth yet this activity ended up severely wounding my mouth. Dressing myself is a very long, and tedious, process. I recall once I woke up at 5 A.M. just to be ready by 8:00. I was exhausted and didn't have any ambition to do much of anything all that day.

There's so much about my own physical limitation that I don't understand and, as years go pass, I find that my inability to achieve many activities intensifies! When I was young, I would strive to be as 'normal' as the people around me were. It wasn't till later on in my life that I figured out that each being born on this earth has some form of an affliction! What's normal? For years you modeled yourself after someone you thought 'had it all together' yet, somehow, you failed. That's what I did for so many years. Ann J. helped me to realize that I could not be like anyone else. I had to form my own abilities into what I can do, instead of what will never transpire.

I passed the first and second grades in the first of five years at Ann J. As I said before, I was a smart brat for my age and I astonished all the teachers I ever had. This society has a false concept that assumes, since your body doesn't function up to their expectations, then your mind's worthless! Mr. Perry was my third grade teacher. Nothing spectacular occurs during this year. I learned that the odd numbered grades can be harder than the even numbered grades. I must have had all my real hair back, by then, because I never looked like a two-eyed bowling ball again. Mrs. Plumber was my forth, fifth and sixth grade teacher. You know how kids get strange notions in their heads. Well, I was no different! For the longest time I thought Mrs. Plumber was originally a plumber. She was very nice, and always had faith in me that I could do anything that I set my mind to!

September of 1964 brought many new and different experiences. I arrived at Ann J. to start my fifth grade when this black lady met me at the door and rolled me to my locker. While she helped me off with my jacket, she told me her name was Mrs. Owens and she'd be my staff from then on. This was the first time I had worked with a person of a different race and we became best of friends. I never could figure out why Dad always refered to them as 'Niger's', as if they should be punished for being born African-American. Mrs. Owens would meet me at the door, took my coat off and made sure I didn't need the restroom. Then, she took me around to my daily appointments and fed me a good lunch. I would always remember coming into school, just after New Year's of 1965, and telling her that I turned into a woman the night before.

"I'm bleeding, Mrs. Owens!" I said sheepishly.

"What do you mean?" She asked.

"Well, I woke up this morning and my bed was all bloody! It scared me for a minute and then Mom told me I began my menstrual cycle. Oh, Mrs. Owens, I have a stomach-ache!" I was about in tears.

"Oh honey, you're just having cramps. That's normal. It only lasts around four days and comes once a month. This is so that you can have babies when you get older. It's best to keep yourself busy so that you don't think about the pain."

She took my coat off and rolled me into Mrs. Plumber's room. Little did I realize but every month Mom got mad at me for having periods. There were times when she threatened to have me fixed because, she claimed, no man could ever love me! I never knew about sex, at that time, yet I always wanted to be in love! I figured this was a way Mom released some of her frustrations.

Bus #23 was my school bus for five years. I memorized that routes until I knew it backwards and could tell the drivers, who substituted when our regular driver was sick, the right streets to turn on. I always had to sit in the front seat, which wasn't cool for any kid to do, because Mom had to carry me up those narrow stairways that all buses had. I say it wasn't cool because you couldn't get away with much when you sat in the first three seats! The driver would spot any mischief through his rear view mirror. Besides, all the cute boys sat in the back of the bus! When Mom would take me for sunny, afternoon drives; I would proudly point out the streets that bus #23 drove down.

During my third year of riding bus #23, I became good friends with a blind girl by the name of Alicia. As a matter of fact, she had a twin sister whose name was Tabitha. Alicia once told me that, when they were born, both only weighed two ounces. You could hold them in the palm of your hand. One was so shy while the other was quite a talker. I recall Alicia's head was constantly moving, as if she had a built in radio in her brain. They taught me a lot about seeing life without using your eyes. Alicia would describe the beauty of the sunrise and teach me how tender the tips of their fingers were. They did their homework by Braille and saw this world with the precious gift that only comes from the heart.

"The people on the bus go up and down! Up and down! Up and down, all the way to school!" That was the old children's song I used to sing to myself to pass the time away while our bus traveled all around the suburbs of Battle Creek. I had a low volume voice and really had to articulate each word in order to be understood. Hardly anyone could hear my goose-like singing, so I would sit there and imagine myself as a thin Mama Cass or a white Diana Ross.

I recall a fellow, who was in the ninth grade that always made his way to the back of the bus. Chuck was his name and, every time he got on the bus, I silently prayed that he would stop at my seat. I found out later that he had a French girlfriend who he was planning on going over to see as soon as he graduated from high school. I felt a rise each time he crept up to my seat as the bus was nearing his house. Once, when the bus was almost empty, Chuck serenaded me with a song that was big in 1967. He sang, "What the World Needs Now is Love Sweet Love!" That gave me a thrill for days after that.

Ann J. Kellogg's elementary school was five years of discoveries. Five years of developing skills, of opening my self up and experiencing much of the reality of life which is essential for growth. Of gaining friendships that would last forever! You must realize a human being's existence on this earth is like a rose bush. A rose bush must have a firm foundation. Rich soil, sunlight, rain, and time for growth. In the same process, a human life requires opportunities to develop and mature in order to become all that God intended a soul to be. Ann J. and Northwestern Junior High enabled me to continue this conversion.

Northwestern Junior High was my first experience with normalcy. That was years ago yet, to this very day, I cannot figure out what's 'normal' and what's not? This was where I found out how cruel my 'so called' peers could be towards wheelchair people. For example, in my homeroom science class, Mrs. B. asked if anyone would take notes, for me, with carbon paper. No one raised his or her hand. I had to sit in the back of her classroom, and almost had to buy a telescope to see over the heads of my fellow classmates. Mrs. B. was public enemy #1 with any kid in the whole school. She ended up using the carbon paper to take notes for me! Mrs. B. was strict, yet had to be in order to getting her point across. I recall a day in 1968, where the black kids of the school rebelled against discrimination. That was a big issue of that time and, since Mrs. B. was already on their 'hit list' for giving hard exams, they marched to her homeroom to 'sit in'. I was scared. Isn't it funny how life goes in cycles? I was frightened by a sector of our society who was discriminated in all areas of their lives. They had to sit in back of buses, refrain from using the 'white man's' restrooms and many other ridiculous rules, which must have made the black population feel less than human.

Mrs. B.'s classroom was next door to a handsome hunk of God's creation. Mr. K. was his name and, having my homeroom next door to his, gave me a legitimate reason to peek in his door on my way to and from class. I caught a glimpse of this gorgeous blue eyed blond at least once a day. When I heard that he was a karate expert on the side, I used to pray that he would cut a block of wood for me. Then, it happened! I remember the day he called me into his room and split a four by four with his bare hands for me. I slept with that piece for days after that.

I remember once I had a crush on my seventh grade math teacher. I mean he made my soul do flip-flops every time he looked my way during class. He asked anyone in the class if they knew an answer to this one problem and I got very excited. I thought, "Now, I will show him I do have brains!" At that time, I had to constantly hold my head up by tightly grasping the right side of my chair. I forgot I had one of my death grips on my chair and began to raise my right hand. Well, to my embarrassing surprise, the whole right side of my chair came off. Man, I could have died right there and then. I answered the question anyway like nothing had happened.

I looked at my yearbook today and wondered who married whom? Wouldn't it have been nice to be on the top of one of those human pyramids? I went on my first 'date' on January 8, 1968. A boy named Tim escorted me to one of our school basketball games, and during halftime we rode up the halls exhibiting our friendship to the teachers who were working late. I thought I was so 'cool' to have someone take an interest in me. Little did I know that the spring of 1968 would be the last time I would actually be attending an institute of higher learning for fourteen years.

Chapter 3

The Lonely Years

"She has none to comfort her. Among all her lovers, all her friends have dealt treacherously with her. They have become her enemies."

Lamentations; 1-2

I spent three-fourths of my day on the floor. I remember August 8, 1968 as a day that will endure forever. I got tired of doors slamming, which only meant I was alone again. I really needed someone to talk to. Someone who would never walk away or treat me like some useless piece of furniture! On this August afternoon, I was playing on my bedroom floor when I suddenly looked up at my crucifixes that hang over my bed. I recall hearing that each person on earth must have a personal relationship with Christ. I said my first prayer to Him directly, and not to the Holy Mother. I felt I needed to keep Mom happy and so I still did my rosary yet knew now I had a direct line to the main Man!

I recall the time Mom sat me outside my bedroom window. There was a young tree standing with his branches toward the sky as if he was praising the Lord for another spring day. I forgot Mom was cleaning my room, with the window open, and began vocalizing my thoughts to God.

"Who are you talking to?" Mom glanced out the screen.

I looked around and all I could think to answer was, "The tree, It looks lonely."

Mom just smiled and went back to work. Does it really matter if my life stems from an electric wheelchair? Satan had a field day at my birth many years ago yet this doesn't indicate that I'm any less of a woman. I have physical and emotional disorders, like any other lady, before my menstruation. My cravings and desires for lovers and friends are not terminated just because I have severe Cerebral Palsy. This society tends to be blind to the fact that, no matter what physique anyone has, they still need to express their own identity!

Then came a season of my life where I felt the most imprisoned by my physical disability. My parents found out my pea brain certainly does hold an enormous amount of knowledge, yet the trick would be to reveal to society that I am much more than a couch potato. I had my idols like everyone else! For the longest time I thought Neil Diamond was just waiting for me to grow up so we could get married! I recall the Association and the Fifth Dimension were just so 'groovy'. The Monkeys had one of my favorite songs that became my theme song. "I want to be free, like the blue bird flying by me..." Yes, the radio was my best friend! I loved the Mamas and Papas and thought it was so 'cool' to be fat, as well as famous, both at once!

We moved to a suburb of Battle Creek, called Harper Creek in 1968. It gave Dad more elbowroom, yet put me in a secluded situation. We lived on six and a half-mile road across from a cow field. I recall each fall they would take a truckload of heifers to the slaughterhouse. I had a tear in my eye whenever I saw the cows, which gave birth that spring, being lead into this cage-like truck. It reminded me of the holocaust in Germany! There was a large black bull that lived in a field cattycornered from those twelve cows. I used to refer to them as his harem. One June afternoon, this king of the beef kingdom, must had been very horny. He broke away from the chains that bound him to his isolated island and jumped the fence. Well, this fine hunk of prime rib anxiously ran up my road and got caught in our yard. His cow friends were screaming like lost lovers finally finding each other.

Did I ever tell you how I'm writing these words? When I was young, I always wanted to keep a diary but am unable to use my hands. Since dictating isn't very private, Mom and I developed a way I could type by wearing a helmet. That hockey helmet had a wand attached to the front, about seven inches in length, and I peck at the keys I need. If memory serves me right, it was during the year 1970 that we devised that way of communication.

The next eighteen months consisted of a battle between my parents against the Battle Creek School system. The system wanted me to be transported to Central High, which is a three-story building in the "rougher" section of Battle Creek. Our house was only a mile from a one-floor high school. After a two year fight, I finally got permission to be placed on a home bound program where three tutors came to the house three days a week for the next four years.

Each Monday, Wednesday and Friday I had my high school right in my kitchen. Mrs. K. taught math and English. She was a tall thin woman who always made me feel good about myself. Mr. R. taught writing. He was a handsome guy, but he didn't go in detail with writing. You might say, he was a piece of cake. I had Mr. G., who reminded me of a miniature Colombo, for science. Don't get me wrong, Colombo is a man I highly admire. Mr. G. would be constantly thinking yet not much came out of his mouth. I recall the last two weeks of school were the only time, out of the whole year, that he could get the eighteen films that I was required to see for high school.

Mom made popcorn and all three of us sat in the livingroom watching Shakespearean plays, such as Macbeth or Romeo and Juliet, or tiresome narration of the conception of a rutabaga. The life of a bean usually put me to sleep and I ended up glancing out the window daydreaming. None of my three tutors knew algebra or geometry. This was unfortunate because I'm great with numbers.

Mom would write my homework out yet, no matter if I gave the wrong answer, she would put it down. I'll never forget the many nights we wrote out long division. Math was my best subject and we would work at the dining table for two hours at a time.

On June 8, 1974 these three tutors gave me a very official ceremony that lasted eight hours. Mrs. K. held it at her house and I even got to wear a cap and gown. I wanted, so much, for my parents to be there but Dad never liked being around people and Mom didn't feel right going alone. If I remember correctly, Dad was ready for his afternoon nap when Mrs. K.'s husband, Gary, picked me up to go to my graduation.

Mrs. K., and Gary took care of disabled dogs at the time of my graduation. Some of the canines had missing legs while others had only one eye. After I got my diploma, Gary sat me in one of their brown bean bag chairs. It felt as if I was sitting on Jell-O. This was an experience in itself yet, when the dogs found out they could climb on top of me, I was bombarded by dogs. I will never forget that day. It was an unforgettable moment in time that was exciting but sad in knowing none of my own family came.

When I became twenty in 1973, I had a second doctor confirm this theory of my ignorance. Dr. Sanders spent only a half-hour with me, while being interrupted five times by phone calls. Dr. Sanders managed to write a five page report declaring my I.Q. as twenty-nine and accusing Mom of being a liar. The accusation against Mom was over a take home math test, which I was to complete on my own. The only assistance I had from my Mom was writing my answers down for me. Being the honest woman Mom is, she only wrote down my answers whether they were right or wrong. Dr. Sanders had insisted that Mom had taken the test for me and in his wrongful assumptions disregarded her intelligence because it did not agree with his report. I showed that physiologist that he was totally wrong when I graduated with a B average from high school.

During that season of my life, I had none of my peers around me. I found myself lying on our livingroom floor was much of my daily routine, and the radio became my best friend. We started each day with a knock-knock joke from Mr. Moose while Ping-Pong balls were forever bombarding Captain Kangaroo. Once, every three weeks, the Captain would let us view the changing of the guards at Buckingham Palace in England. We learned that these guards aren't allowed to crack a smile while they're on duty or they would loose their jobs. I couldn't handle that! Life's too short not to crack a grin at people who passes me as I'm rolling down a sidewalk! Who knows, I might make somebody's day?

Mom and I would answer questions to game shows all morning, as we did the housework. Mom was seldom wrong and I found much of my eccentric education came from these active times. We would eat lunch over Hollywood Squares and Jeopardy. Charlie Weaver and Paul Lynn were two of our favorite squares. In later years, Hollywood Squares got too risqué for my taste! I had the day's programming memorized better than the TV guide and knew each character as if they were my next door neighbors. Afternoons were spent with four and half-hours of soap operas. Between "Days of our Lives" and "Another World", Mom would knit ten more rows of her latest afghan.

At 3:00 PM., Lynn, Joseph and John came home from school. Lynn would run into her room and five minutes later, come out looking like Annie Oakley.

"How were your classes today, did your calculus exam go ok?" Mom would ask Lynn.

"So, so. Can I take these apple peels out to Smoky?" Smoky was her horse dad gave her for her sixteenth birthday. Lynn would sleep with Smoky if Mom would let her.

The back door slammed as Mom was in the middle of her "Try not to be late for supper." warning.

Joseph would hang his school jacket up in the hall closet and go searching for a big salad bowl that he filled with corn flakes. Then he went into his room, shut the door behind him, and read one of his three thousand science fiction books. Three of his four walls were lined with paperback novels. Mom and I would never see him, or John, again before supper. John would do the same only he would take Fruit Loops and work on his stamp collection.

I would know when 5:00 PM. came for dad arrived through the front door after a hard day of firing people. He seldom talked, and I learned that mental pain is far more damaging than any physical beatings we could experience! Whoever said silence is golden never knew my dad. Mom got it from all sides. If dad had a hard day at work, or it rained on the day he wanted to mow our yard; we would get the silent treatment for days. This came with slamming of doors, and turning up the thermostat up to eighty-five degrees while he ran around the house in his underwear. They never really talked it out, whenever they had problems, except where I was concerned. They never spoke for weeks at a time, and I hardly ever saw them kiss.

I recall dad's first pair of stereo headphones. One year, on Christmas Eve, he stayed up all night eating buttered popcorn, and listening to Beethoven's 9th in stereo. He simply couldn't believe stereo headphones! Both my parents enjoyed classical music, which gave me a deep fascination for Beethoven, Mozart and Chopin. They also liked the big band sound.

I grew up with the Mamas and Papas, Barbara Streisand and Neil Diamond. The '80s' gave me Lionel Richie and Phil Collins to swoon over. Mom loved to play the organ, sometimes by ear. My family was musically inclined and could perform tunes simultaneously without ever reading a note. I would only fool around with the footpedals because I never had much control of my fingers.

Dad would always feed me while mom served the meal as she sat on the other side of the table. Dad had a beer, and half of another, in him by the time supper was ready. I recall Joseph sat on the left side, of dad, while John sat across from him. I learned my French around the table. Mom would ask each of my brothers for items, such as salt, but she would ask in French. On the evenings we had beef stew, Joseph would pile everything on his plate together and mix it all up. Then he would spread all of it between two slices of bread. Meanwhile, John would make sure his carrots did not touch his potatoes and each different food had its rightful place on his plate.

We fail to realize that fame and material possessions won't hold you tight on a lonely night! Many believe sex is the answer to any problem that crosses their path. It might feel good all through a night yet, when morning comes, you're back to facing this bitter reality unaccompanied. I never really knew Dad's favorite food, or his philosophy on life. Never recalled him saying, "I love you" to any of us, or found out what gave him the most happiness. I had many opportunities to talk to him. He invited me out to sit in the back yard to watch the grass grow or pick dandelions for dandelion wine. We never really talked. Dad always had a beer or a glass of gin as he staggered around the garden pulling weeds. In the spring and summer all he wore was a white T-shirt and long pants.

By noontime this shirt would be a dirty, grayish garment holding three hours worth of perspiration when he would finally go indoors to turn on a baseball game. Once again, around 1 PM., Dad was snoring away either on the livingroom couch or sprawled on the floor beside the TV. As the afternoon ran on, snores grew louder than the announcer on the screen did.

Dad would wake up during the eighth inning and start drinking again. The one neighbor we had, on Six and a Half-Mile Road, would watch him stumble over his own feet as Dad's stomach lapped excessively beyond his belt. There were times when his pants began to fall down. This was very embarrassing to watch yet no one could tell Dad anything. He was hiding within a glass bottle and it's extremely hard to talk to a person through the glass! This occurred every weekend. He never really knew me, as I sat watching the gin take effect, Dad talked at me until he was lost within himself.

Mom would do the weekly grocery shopping on Saturday mornings. Dad never liked being around other people, after coming home from his government job at 5:00 each weeknight, so Mom had to attend PTA meetings and all social events alone. She needed to talk, but never felt comfortable going out unaccompanied. After all, she was married and society expects a married couple to be together in all activities. She needed friends! She needed those brief periods where she got away from the house. Time for her self and a pause from taking care of me! The one to four hours, that mom was away; dad had to take care of me. These were the most frightening intervals of my life. It might not have been so bad if dad wasn't drunken three-fourths of the time. If I had to use the bathroom, he would take me. If you can picture a drunken man trying to balance a spastic Cerebral Palsy child, who was born without any equilibrium, you can see why I feared dad watching me.

Well, I had some relief when Jerry C. asked me to work on a committee for the physically disabled of Battle Creek. The minute Jerry would come, to pick me up for a meeting, dad would quickly stumble back to his bedroom. After all, he spent fifty percent of his time in his underwear! It felt very awesome to be working along side Jerry knowing all to well that I was once a student of his. As I think back, I would had confided in Jerry more yet I was young and thought parents could do no wrong. Jerry would transfer me in his car and away we drove. This made me feel very important. I recall one cold November evening. Jerry wanted to promote our wheelchair-bowling league and so he called me, and asked if I would pose for some shots for our local newspaper. Dad wouldn't take me to the alley so Jerry offered to pick me up. Well, being physically transferred into a car has its advantages, especially when a handsome hunk does it. One November evening, as Jerry was helping me out, my feet landed on a chuck of ice and I slid under the car.

"Hey, where do you think you're going?" He looked down at me. "Oh, as long as you are down there, will you check my oil?" He smiled, as he carefully lifted me back into my chair.

Jerry was the type of person, who did a hundred percent of his job and two hundred percent more. He treated me like any other person he knew. His dad was our coach for our bowling team. We bowled on ramps that reminded me of mini roller coasters. I remember how excited I got when I rolled my very first ball. I had one of my spastic fits and threw the ball so vigorously that the ball actually hopped into the next lane. Jerry's dad promised each one of us a turkey if we got three strikes in a row. We had fun! We were each needed and felt as if we belonged! During 1971, Jerry's dad became very ill and died around New Year's of '72'. I have never felt like bowling since then. It's not the same game anymore.

Grandpa Schauder died in that same year. Dad went down to stay with him for a week. Dad thought his condition was improving so he came back to Battle Creek. Three days later, around 5:00 A.M., the phone rang. Everyone seemed to be awake for some reason. Dad came into the back porch, which was my bedroom at that time, and sat down beside me and cried. Grandpa had past away earlier that morning.

Mom knew I needed someone to talk to so she called Big Brothers and Big Sisters. It was a chilly November evening when Dorothy became a friend who is still my best friend today. She started coming once a week to play cards or watch movies. She got married to a man named Gary, who worked where dad worked. He's a car lover and a tease. Just recently retired, they are both enjoying traveling and collecting car parts.

One of Dad's co-workers told him about a facility for physically disabled people. I never belonged in a home, so my parents requested an interview with Reverend Brown, the executive director of Echoing Hills Residential Center. In the beginning, he had a vision! A dream of having a summer camp for multi-handicapped individuals. The camp started in 1966, but then Reverend Brown saw that there was a need for somewhere these physically challenged people could have an environment they could call home. On June 10, 1973, Echoing Hills Residential Center opened its doors to nine people who now felt they had a place to hang their hat.

Dave J. drove up to our house, because he knew the highways better than Reverend Brown did. Dave was the director of the camp, which is on the same grounds, but a totally different feature of Echoing Hills. Reverend Brown had Cerebral Palsy, yet his type permitted him to be ambulatory. Reverend Brown drives and even tells bad jokes, as well as being a reverend. Mr. Brown said I was a perfect candidate for his 20-bed home. In today's lingo you could say, "I was the right stuff." It was amazing to see dad stay around for the whole interview. He was never much for company. He would normally run and hide when the doorbell rang.

It's strange what death can do? In October 1976 a man by the name of Ed P. passed away from a heart attack. He was one of the first residents to live there, when the home opened up on June 10, 1973. I didn't have that much to think over. Feeling that I was chaining mom down, like some wild palomino longing to be free from the rope that binds her, I prayed beside the back door of my bedroom. So much raced through my mind! I never seen Echoing Hills, yet, this move would free mom to do what she wanted with her own life. I finally agreed, and, on April 1, 1977, dad loaded me into the car for the seven and a half-hour ride down to Warsaw Ohio. I remember John, my youngest brother, coming out and watching our parents me drive away. He cried! This was the first time, in my life, that I knew that he cared about me! I had tears in my eyes.

Chapter 4

Echoing Hills

"The Lord shall preserve thy going out and thy coming in from this time forth, and even for nevermore."

Psalm 121:8

A woman has to do what has to be done! An abundance of happenings occurred during this span of time. Various good friendships sprinkled with a few passionate love affairs and far too many partings. I even grew three inches in ten days.

On the first day I found out that there were two married couples living here. Jerry and Barb E. both had Cerebral Palsy. Don and Sue were the other couple. Sue also had Cerebral Palsy, whereas her husband had Polio. I recall meeting Don and Sue T. in the dining room and Don had a really gross way of introducing his friends who sat around him to me.

"Here's my better half, Sue!" He nodded his head towards Sue. "And then we have Bill M. we refer to him as BM." Everyone snickered.

I thought "What a way to be remembered!"

Nearly half my life, I fooled myself by thinking that, to be totally happy during this mortal experience, one must follow a series of events which society claims you need to have a fulfilling existence! Well, guess what? I finally learned that this concept is all wet! My life-style can never live up to yours, yet, why should it? It's insane to model your time on this earth after anyone's but our Lord Jesus Christ!

22

Anyway, getting back to the 'gang', I met my first roommate shortly after midnight on April 1, 1977. Pat was her name and, ten of the residents were just getting back from Florida. She had Cerebral Palsy, like Reverend Brown, was ambulatory. For a brief moment, I thought I was in a Co-ed dorm.

An orderly, by the name of Rod, was escorting her to our room. They both sounded as if they had one too many. Of course, everyone gets giddy when they are exhausted. As for me, I hid under my covers until I knew the guy wasn't staying there. I remember Pat trying very hard to whisper but to no avail. I was as eager to get to know who was my roommate as she was excited to know how much of the gossip was true about me.

Pat was just beginning a new life as a divorcee. I never met anyone who had Cerebral Palsy and, had been married, let alone divorced. Pat and I became more like sisters than roommates. She had a crazy infatuation over the bread man when she worked at the Post. The Post was our corner store. I remember he made weekly deliveries and, she would wear her best perfume on those days. She ran the cash register and, I always referred to him as her "Wonder Man!"

At one time we were fighting over the same boyfriend. Paul A. was his name and he lifted weights for a hobby. He had Cerebral Palsy, and like Pat, walked with a spastic shake. Whenever he ate, he poured ketchup over his food, and placed everything on his plate into sandwich form. This was so that he could feed himself everything at once. The ketchup was mainly because he was Italian, besides adding flavor to many of the foods that they served there. Paul had muscles on top of muscles, which might be why he was the 'Casanova' of the home at one time. Once, Pat even pulled my hair because Paul was taking an interest in me. Nothing ever happened between Paul and I. Pat and I remain friends to this day.

June G. was our main cook at that time. There were twenty-seven residents when I first came and we all called her 'Mom'. Her husband, Harry, owned the Post back then. It was a small corner store at the beginning of Echoing Hills long driveway. Harry was seventeen years older than June was. June really made each one of us feel like just another one of her kids. She had a special liking towards Paul, and for mother's day each year, he would buy her twelve long stem roses. He knew which side his bread was buttered on!

I just found a bag of letters that Mom kept for so many years. I never realized she had these and find them very informative plus valuable to the writing of this book. The first letter is the beginning of my pen-palship to my mother from Echoing Hills. It goes like this...

4/3/77

Dear Mom,

I miss you! I hope you and Dad got back OK? The people here are very nice. My roommate's name is Pat; too, so some nurses call me Clam, my last name sounds like chowder. We had a big dinner today but it wasn't like Dad's. We had chicken, peas, mash-potatoes and apple stuff. By the time I got to eat, most of my food was cold. They had three tables and the nurses dish up everyone's plate. We had breakfast at 8:15, lunch at 12:15 and supper at 5:15. I miss your cooking very much.

They are saying Pat and I might have to move into a smaller room. Actually, every other room is bigger than ours is. I went around and saw that, compared to ours, most residents had more room. I hoped I didn't move until I get my own room.

I couldn't go to church today because Reverend Brown is still driving the bus back from Florida. Tomorrow I'm meeting all the big wheels. I'm kind-of nervous about that. I think I'm going to love it here, even if I miss you a lot. I won't get my TV set up for two weeks. I was lucky to get a shelf up Friday. It's small but I got six music boxes and five picture things on it.

I knew it would be strange at first, yet, I don't know why I still cry a bit. It's everything I wanted and more. I will be OK once I get busy.

Last night I bumped my head. I'm better today. I hope you're feeling a little better. I'm getting up by 8:00 A.M. every morning and in bed by 11:30 PM. Easter morning we have a service up on the hill at 7:00 A.M. I hope it won't be too windy. Well, Happy Easter! Tell everyone hi. I miss you all!

4/4/77

Dear Dad and Mom,

How are you? It's raining today and I have a small cold. The nurse started me on Penicillin pills. My throat is really red but I'm feeling pretty good other than that.

I really am getting to like this place. I could use a new bedspread. The one I have now is very dull. I put on my new sheets today, and they look very nice. I think I could use around twenty-five dollars, because we're going shopping on the 23rd. I had to pay seven dollars and fifty cents in July it's for the resident's fund. We're having a resident's meeting tonight but, since I'm new, I didn't have to pay this.

I love you very much! Tell everyone hi!

4/11/77

Dear Mom,

I miss you very much! How are you? How's everyone? I went to church yesterday, after we had a sunrise service down in a building on the campgrounds. Six other residents go to the same church as I do. It's a large church, and the people are nice. I met Sister Claire who comes out here sometimes. She's tall, yet, doesn't look like a Sister. I wore my pink outfit, and Uncle Jim sent me a flower. I looked nice, believe it or not!

I'm almost over my cold, but six other residents have it now! I started feeding myself, without my feeder, and it seems to be going OK. I'm using my left hand and I like it better than my right. I arranged a bake sale for May 21st, and everyone liked my memo. Next Saturday, we're going to a wedding. The man who came up with Reverend Brown is getting married. I may get to go to Carol's wedding in August. The great thing about it is you and Dad doesn't have to help me get there. They have a guestroom where you can stay and spend a few days here. I still cry for you and Dad, yet, I really think I'll like it here.

5/3/77

Dear Mom,

I miss you! Happy Mother's Day! I wish I could get you something. In fact, I feel sorry that I can't get the most beautiful Mom in the world something. I'll be thinking of you Sunday. [Not to mention all week, every day of the week]

I got your letter today and you sound good. I also got Uncle Jim's. I haven't opened it yet. Tomorrow, I'm seeing a psychiatrist. David said they didn't want any more of my back history. I hope he's better than Mrs. Dickinson. Everyone says all the girls swoon over him. I'm kind-of nervous but you know me. I got my tires today, but they aren't on my chair yet. I'm going for my interview Friday, at the TV station, and now I know I'll go in my electric wheelchair.

Well I better go now. Have a nice Sunday and keep up your typing. Keep smiling! I think you better send away for more shoes for me. My old white pair already has a hole in the toe.

5/20/77

Dear Mom,

How are you? I have been very busy or, it has been too hot to type. It has been eighty and over for the last few days. Last Friday, I got four large print books and I'm half way done with one. I'm so behind in my personal letters that I didn't know if I would ever catch up.

I went to a physical therapy evaluation and I have a lot more work to do. I have PT a half-hour in the morning and a half-hour in the afternoon. I will do sit-ups, push-ups, sitting on the edge of the mat, by myself, and working out with weights. I had to buy some better shoes because, the kind I had weren't good for transferring. I was going shopping on their monthly shopping spree. I also have to spend half the day in my manual chair, which I don't like but they want me to use more muscles.

I got those two Lettermen tapes yesterday. I like them, even if they don't sing "Feelings" very well. We are going to a fair on the fourth. I had planned to take my roommate out to dinner on the fourth. The fair will take all day. I'm going to take her out on the 11th with two other people. Pat birthday is June 2nd; yet, she has plans for that evening. I keep telling her that we are going shopping so she won't know. Are you still coming down in June? Dot wrote that she's coming in the last part of June. I only hope you come to that contest in August. By the way, I need that fifty dollars entry fee, or, did you want me to take it out from downstairs?

We moved our beds around in our room and, now it looks a little bigger. I have your picture turned so I can see you when I wake up. I'll never stop missing you. I wish you didn't live *so far away. I don't mind being at Echoing Hills, even if it is frightening not having anyone around who really knows and understands me. I miss you and Dad but, I'm making it OK. Tell everyone hi! Could you send me some tank tops?*

5/29/77

Dear Mom and Dad,

Happy Memorial Day! I hope you are all fine. Last night, I called you, because I was down all day. I got Hell from, at least, three people. I was going on an all day trip, yet I couldn't go because they said I changed my mind too much. We have a new program director and, this was the first minor outing she had. Everything went like the Cerebral Palsy group outings go up there. I got all upset because, I was all set to go and then I didn't. I went back into the home when, one of my fellow residents' got me in trouble.

Debbie's her name and, she would get anyone in trouble if she wants to. In fact, we all may be grounded and, have to stay in our rooms because, some money has been taken from her roommate. Once, before I came, seventy dollars was taken and, everyone had to stay in their rooms and, were not allowed to play tapes or TV or anything till the money was found. It turned out to be Debbie who took it.

I talked to Mrs. Bailey after I talked to Dad last night. I had been hearing a lot of rumors about this place that frighten me. I guess I'm still adjusting and, once I get in college, my whole life will be better. Everyone tells me things and, it's hard to know whom to trust right now. I'm mixed-up yet, It will take time to be real happy here. Everyone says get out when you can so, Wednesday night I'm going out to dinner. Saturday, I want to take my roommate out for her birthday.

I guess I called Dad when I was in a down mood. I didn't know whom to turn to. I'm sorry for calling twice in one week, yet, I'm happier when I talk to you and Dad. I decided, if you can wait, don't come down in June. We are going shopping on the

11th and, Dot might come down later in June. I think it will be better if you waited. I love you so much but, I need time to grow.

Anyway, I'm concentrating now on my body more than my mind. I sit in my manual everyday till noon or 1:00PM. I push myself around and, in PT I did twenty sit-ups on Friday. My new shoes are working better for transfers but my left foot is giving me trouble because of my toes.

I woke up happy but then, during devotions, John told us Friday would be his last day. Last Monday Mr. Kale fired him because John told him what was wrong about something. I have grown close to John and his family so, I cried. I mean, there aren't many people that I can talk to when I'm down. I will really miss him. Rod said I could go into town with him to buy John a going away gift. Rod also said they're firing a lot of good people, which scares me. Once, Mr. Kale told the staff that they should have good relationships with the residents but, after we do, he fires them. I don't understand. Anyway, John had to walk out even before we said grace because he was beginning to cry.

I got Mr. Campbell's 8-track tape last Saturday. I must have played it twenty times by now. My roommate likes it more than I thought she would. Today, if it doesn't rain, we're going swimming and having a cook out. Then, we'll go on a hayride. I love hayrides!

I opened up a bank account last week with ninety dollars. I like it yet, now I don't want to take fifty dollars out for my entry fee for that contest. I just put it in Friday.

I saw the doctor last Wednesday and I need some tests and an X-ray. I spent two hours waiting for him, in my room, and he spent only ten minutes with me! Boy, I didn't like waiting around.

7/2/77

Dear Mom,

How are you? Happy 4th of July! I'm writing this in the middle of an earache. I don't know what happened, but I was lying outside and at 4:30 PM. it began to bug me. I told David, the nurse that's on tonight, and he said it's red. He gave me some eardrops. I was planning to go to church tomorrow but, now I'm staying home.

I hope it clears up by Monday because we're going to the fair grounds to have a picnic and see the fire works. I think I'll wear my three-piece outfit. We'll start out at 2:00 PM. and be home by 10:00 PM.

Either Wednesday or Friday Tommie, Jane, Karen and I will go shopping for my formal dress for Miss Wheelchair of Ohio. I'm taking around seventy dollars out of the bank in order to get a good formal and a pair matching of shoes. I'm so happy that you and Dad are coming. It means a lot to me. This is something I never dreamt of doing and, I want the two people, who I love very much, to be there. I got your reservations ready for the 20th. They sent me a map of where it's going to be and, Karen made me a copy to send to you. I only hope I make you proud of me. I'll do my best! Thanks for coming.

I believe I was one of the five finalists in that competition. I wore a dark pink gown and my first pair of dress shoes. I was so proud of myself. One of my roommates, Dee, became one of the five finalists also, but in the year 1978.

10/30/77

Dear Mom,

How are you? We had our library done, and it's very nice. They made one long table for typewriters, with shelves behind the typewriters for personal books and things. That is where I'm typing this letter. This library is in the basement, and somehow I would love to stay here till bedtime.

Tomorrow the state inspectors are coming, and everyone's either uptight, or going in circles, or mad at certain people. I hate it when state people come; everything has to be professional. We had to have only two cups on the sink and our soap. Everything else has to be out of sight. I feel like I'm in a zoo. Half of our staff either got fired or quit in the last two weeks so we're really mixed-up. Mr. Kale said we can move into the new part in three weeks, but somebody told me that the nurse's station wouldn't be done before December 1st.

Friday night, we had a pumpkin carving party, which was OK. We sang stupid Halloween carols such as, "I'm dreaming of the Great Pumpkin." I didn't feel good anyway. Last night, some of us went on a hayride. We went up to Reverend Brown's for a Halloween party. I was Sherlock Holmes. All the people I like to be with stayed at the home. Some of my favorite staff were there.

Well, it's after supper, about 5:30 PM., and I just had the last of my milk since I was still full from dinner. I didn't feel like going to church, so I slept until 9:30 A.M. Tommie and I both thought it was 10:30 A.M. but after we got up, we remembered the time change.

I might be going with Laura, a staff, to surprise a few camp counselors next weekend. Denise is coming from Florida for three days, and we thought we would take her to Columbus, and surprise some more counselors.

Tommie's going to Florida next Sunday, which means I will have the room to myself for a week. After she comes back, she plans on spending a week in the hospital. She'll take my electric wheelchair, because she won't have to be pushed then. I have the room to myself half of November also.

11/10/77

Dear Mom,

How are you? Did you go back to work? I hope you did. I know how Dad can get on your nerves. I found out that I might be allergic to chocolate. Last Friday, I treated myself to chocolate mints, and then I took my shower. I broke out all down my back, and around my neck. It's strange because all summer we thought Tommie was allergic to chocolate, and here it might be me.

This has been a very busy week, since two of the hardest residents went to Florida. [I mean hard to handle] I guess eighteen of the twenty residents, who went, are total care people. I'm very glad I didn't go because of that and other problems that they are having. Tommie is the only one with an electric wheelchair, which means many of the staff, are pushing two chairs. To add to the whole mess, one of the buses broke down. They're having so many problems that we are praying everyday for them to come back safe. I hope God has a big ear.

I asked Dan P. for my recorder back. He said he would give it back Monday. Boy, does he make me mad! Monday, all he could do was pick his teeth during my class time. Tuesday night, I was fifteen minutes late for class, because I started to feed myself dinner. I forgot about the time so he gave me a small lecture. I gave it right back, and told him that if he could pick his teeth on my time, I could be late once. After all, I'm trying my best to eat by myself. Last night, I almost ate all my dinner without a staff next to me. It was unbelievable because we had mash-potatoes and I found a way of getting them to my mouth.

It's so wonderful, all the things God is showing me. I'm doing more each day. God has been good to me! I have been

35

praying for you and Dad. Last Saturday, Laura took Paul and me to a revival. We're all trying to get Paul closer to God. We started out at 5:30 P.M. and picked up a lady who worked here this summer, then went to the revival. They had some singers and a very good speaker. He spoke on the fear of things and guilt. He almost frightened me, the way his voice cried out his words. I guess Paul liked him. I think he's slightly mixed-up, which, I pray we can help him with. Paul's opening up more, and people are saying it's partly because I'm here. After the revival, we had a good time, even if we didn't get home till midnight.

Next Saturday, we're going on a Christmas shopping spree in Columbus. I don't know if I should go. I went and bought dinner, for a friend, and then I saw a music box that I just had to have. Well, who can turn down Chopin?

I got a bill for the X-ray on my knee. Boy, I never thought pictures could cost so much. I'm waiting till Jane comes back from Florida before doing anything about it.

We elected a new president. Dan N. won eighteen to nine. It was good because, as soon as Dan heard that he won, he went over and shook Jerry's hand.

Well, it seems like everyone's going home for Thanksgiving. It looks like snow tonight. Have a happy holiday.

12/5/77

Dear Dad,

How are you? I got your letter today, and had to thank you and Mom for the money. Yesterday, when we came up from the retreat, I read Mom's letter and was surprised to hear from you so soon after you called. I love both of you very much! I wish we could be together for Christmas, but the Lord must not want it to be. My heart will be with all five of you all through this season.

I can't believe all the beautiful things that God is doing in my life. I had a long talk with the speech teacher [Dan P.], and he isn't as nice as Jerry Campbell yet he is doing a lot for us. I like him now.

We were all moved and have eight new residents. We have thirty-five people at Echoing Hills. Take care of Mom

4/13/78

Dear Mom and Dad,

　　　We had a beautiful Valentine's dinner out. I wore that outfit you gave me for Christmas. I wish you could have seen me. Just before we left, Jim gave me a corsage of yellow and white daisies. I never expected it. I was so happy that I almost cried.

　　　We went to the Blue Drummer, which is a newly opened steak house. When I finally got my food, it was 7:30 PM. Jim saved me a place beside him and Pete Bailey. It was fun. Then Bailey went to eat his own meal while Jim and I talked. I met his Mom and two of his sisters when they brought him back from a weekend visit home. His Mom is beautiful but not as beautiful as you are. Jim can't wait to meet you, Mom and Dad. We talk about you a lot.

　　　Yesterday, we had a counselor from Ohio University of Zanesville come and talk. I enjoyed listening to her. I want to expand my interest by taking at least two classes. I could get more money, from a grant, if I took six or more hours.

　　　Last night, we had our counseling group. We got into a discussing of families. We thought about how some parents have trouble understanding and accepting the new life we are making for ourselves. Jerry and Barb had problems convincing her parents that she can feed herself.

5/8/78

Dear Mom,

How are you? I miss you very much! Happy Mother's Day! I pray you'll have a great Sunday. You're the greatest Mom a girl ever had! I hope you had a safe ride down. I cried when you went, but they were tears of happiness, most of them were. How do the boys like South Carolina? I hope the weather has been better than it has been here. It's been gray and rainy for five days running. I hope it stops by Friday.

Friday, we start our weekend retreat. I will enjoy this one better than the last because it's warmer. This retreat is called the "Kiss Me" retreat. Our cook, June, keeps kidding me by saying that we have to kiss a frog. I will miss sleeping in on Saturday but that's life!

Since it has been raining, I've been working on my novel. I'm using that long green paper and, so far, I have three pages filled. It's about a lady who meets all kinds of people on this elevator. I'm having fun writing it.

We're going to a play Thursday. One of our cook's husbands is in it. We won't be home till midnight. I hope I am alive Monday after I do everything this weekend.

5/22/78

Dear Mom and Dad,

Happy Anniversary! How are you? I just got done with PT, where I did twenty-five sit-ups, and balanced on the edge of the mat. I ache, after last night's walk. I walked for an hour, starting from my room and going all the way down to the dinning room. Then, I got a drink, and walked back to my room. Boy, was I tired!

Saturday night, some of us went to the Miss Wheelchair of Ohio pageant. Dee, our representative, won Miss Achievement, and got in the top five finalists. It was very exciting. We didn't get back till 1:00 A.M. I was still tired from that a week after we came rolling home.

6/19/78

Dear Mom,

How are you? I walked to dinner last night, ate in the walker, and then walked back to my room. I almost didn't make it back, but I took my time and made it. My right foot has been giving me problems so I had it X-rayed last week. I found out, later, that nothing was wrong. It must be the weather.

I love those sundresses. Saturday, just for fun, I went in a dress shop and priced sundresses. The lowest was fourteen dollars, but they didn't look as good as yours. I want a bright yellow one, maybe long, for a wedding.

I might take a trip on the 11th. I owe myself a small vacation, and this will be the first time. Karen the activity coordinator wants to see if I can plan a trip and enjoy it at the same time. I will pray about it. If it's Christ Will, I will go.

The barber's here, and I might get my bangs trimmed. My hair's growing out nicely and I don't think I'll ever cut it short again. Is Dad OK? He seemed down yesterday, over the phone. I'm glad you moved south. I want both of you to be happy. How is your job? Don't work too hard! Take care of yourself.

7/27/78

Dear Mom,

How are you? I can't thank you enough for the box of clothes. I got them today, and said a silent thank you to God for creating such a beautiful Mom as you! I love the clothes, but not as much as I love you. I will write Aunt Ruth, and thank her for the material, but it might not be right away.

I'm very nervous about the C. P. Olympic games, which are a week from Saturday. The residents, who are competing, are going up the night before, because it's a two and a half-hour ride. Karen felt with that long of a trip, we better start around 7:00 PM. Friday evening and sleep at the college where we'll be playing. The residents who will cheer us on will come down Saturday morning. The games start at 9:00 A.M. and go until 5:00 PM. We will go out to dinner after the games, to celebrate, and come home by midnight. Please pray for me, for I'm doing this for the Lord. If I win anything, it'll be for His glory. I'm very excited because yesterday I swam two and a half laps of our pool. We will be swimming twenty-five yards, which is one and one-fifth longer than our pool.

I remember it took me ten minutes and twenty-five seconds to do that lap. The reason why so long is because I was swimming against a current. The main thing is, I never gave up! The next year, I won second place in swimming. I guess it helps when you don't swim against a current. My chair died going up a ramp, which was in the Slalom, yet I ran through it in four minutes and twenty-eight seconds. We came home that year with seventy-seven ribbons.

During this time in my life, my faith in God grew stronger, mainly because I became more independent and active. I realized that my spirituality was changing, however I did not realize to what extent. Looking back on these letters I can see God moving in my life. My new independence caused me to rely on Him more.

Dear Mom,

I just came in from talking with my counselor, and we prayed over some upsetting news. Our cook, Barb, got fired today. She was very good, and worked twelve hours a day sometimes. Barb's getting married to Mrs. Bailey's son. Barb planned to work till the end of August and then quit. That makes two cooks gone within ten days. The odd thing is, we had a staff, named Ruth, who gave her two weeks notice (two weeks ago), but Mr. Kale won't let her go for another week. Ruth makes many of the residents uptight, and mad, besides making more work for the other staff. Yesterday, I went to the doctor almost in tears because of Ruth. God said to accept people the way they are, but it's hard at times.

The doctor said yesterday that my left eye is good, but I have a slight cross-eye in my right. He told me that the cross-eyed came sometime before I became twelve. I can't get any worse, and it's about 20/50. He calls my right eye a lazy eye, but I'm too old to really do anything about it. I can't get any worse than I am now. My glasses are very good, which means I don't need any new lenses. Praise the Lord for that! Psalm 34 talks of praising God at all times. Some of it goes like this...

"1. I will bless the Lord at all times. His praises shall be continually in my mouth. 2. My soul shall make its boast in the Lord. The humble shall hear it and rejoice. 3. O magnify the Lord with me, and let us exalt His name together."

9/16/78

Dear Mom,

How are you? I got your letter today, and wanted to thank you for sending my money, besides I needed to get out of the home. Three-fourths of the residents are watching Ohio State against Penn. State football. You should see the staff and our nurse. I thought Dad was bad, they're three times crazier! Pam, a staff, is more interesting to watch than the game.

Dee loves her dress and couldn't believe it only cost ten dollars. She thanks you and Aunt Ruth very much. I thank you too, for being the world's greatest Mom!

My Bible course is coming along good. I find I'm going all over the Bible instead of just in the book of John. I got rid of some things that Uncle Jim gave me that I didn't want anymore.

Over the phone Dad said that Reverend Brown was going to talk to me about Pat and her mood swings. Dad didn't like hearing about Pat pulling my hair when she found out that her old boyfriend, Paul, was attracted to me. I really doubt he will because he has known her all his life, and I don't think he would say anything against her. I know it's wrong but I can't seem to talk to her anymore. Reverend Brown never discussed Pat with me. It took me awhile to notice the little cliques that are at Echoing Hills. Pat, and Tommie M., were in that circle. I think this was why Tommie became my roommate. As years went by, that circle got more professional and elite.

9/24/78

Dear Mom,

How are you? I got my first two lessons back from my Bible correspondence course, and they both had "A"s on them. I got Tommie's birthday present, and am planning on taking her to dinner on the 4th. It was so great! I was talking to Mr. Kale, and he agreed that we could use the van. Dee and Bill are going also. Pam, and our newest staff Patty, are driving. I feel as if all my prayers are being answered, because very seldom will Kale let us use the van. Tommie's like a sister to me.

Jean C. decided to move back home. I say she's giving up too easy, but she won't listen. Her first college paper got a C, and so she wants to give up on life!

I received an invitation from Dick and Margie Radeloff to come to Don and Wilma's 40th Anniversary. Pam might take me up, and we could visit Uncle Jim the day after the reception. I guess they never had a wedding reception, so Margie is having a surprise reception. I hope I can go. It will be great to see Wilma again. Pam's a very reliable staff.

I heard from Grammy and I wish she could move down by you for the winter. I know God has her in His hands!

10/11/78

Dear Mom,

How are you? I pray for you every day. How is Dad? I really would feel better if you don't try to come up next month. I do want to be near you, on a holiday, but want you safe at home when snow flies. I'm very excited to think that you'll be with me on Thanksgiving, but believe God has a reason for my asking you to stay home.

I went to the dentist yesterday, and I didn't have any cavities. He said that I'll need my wisdom teeth out, in the near future, but I don't know when. I had an appointment on the 20th, to see an orthopedic doctor my back and my foot. I pray that he might have some idea why my foot hurts.!

Dear Mom,

How are you? Last Sunday, we went to the groundbreaking of a new Hill home in Athens. It was windy and cold out, but the ceremony was nice. It'll be next door to a hospital besides being on part of a campus. I don't think I want to move down there, because the state wants seventy-five percent of the residents to come out of state institutions. I'm just settled down here anyway.

Last night, the whole home went to see, "No Longer Alone"'. It was a movie about an English woman who finds Christ. I enjoyed it. I got three more "A's" in my Bible course I can't believe I'm doing this great!

10/21/78

Dear Mom,

Tonight's our last full-body resident meeting of this year. Bill M. won't be running for a second term, and so I doubt if I will stay on the committee after Bill goes. After the meeting, we're having a going away party for one of our nurses. I hate good-byes!

As I told you over the phone, I'm very frightened of this spine operation. I was reading the book, 'Lift up Your Heart' and found out something. God doesn't give us this fear of being afraid. God needs us to face our fears. "We can do all things through Christ who strengthens us." It was odd but after finishing washing my hands, I read part of this book and found that I was reading about the exact feeling that I'm experiencing now! It gave me a good feeling. I know, before I even go to the clinic, they will say it's mandatory to have this operation or someday I won't be able to sit up. I'm praying about it, and the Lord wants me to have it.

Dear Mom,

It's rainy and cold today. After lunch, I'm going into town to vote. I know a little more about the VIPs running than I did last year. Our own election will be next Tuesday. Dee asked me if I would run, but I feel it's a man's job. I could handle the job but, because I might have this operation, I won't have time to do a good job.

I had a crazy dream last night. Dad was about to operate on my back, and you were the nurse. You kept screaming, "No, no, no! Don't do it." I woke up frightened and cried..

1/4/79

Dear Mom,

We had a New Year's Eve party last Sunday night and the theme was Show Biz. Dee came as Diana, of the Supremes, while Sussie and I came as her back up Supremes. We had a bandstand and a dance contest. I was one of the runners up in the twist contest. I never danced so hard in my life. '79' will be a good year!

We're having a winter retreat on the 12th. I'll be glad when it's over. I dislike retreats. I don't know who's excited about them. I'm thinking of going to camp for two weeks in August.

I'm going to Columbus, on the 9th, to see a specialist. I'm slightly nervous but Barb might go with me. I think I know what he'll say, and don't know what Christ wants me to say. I'm praying a lot about next Tuesday and know He will give me the words. I did enjoy the one and half-hours ride over there because we had a new driver, who was very nice. His wife was our newest staff and she was great with us.

1/11/79

Dear Mom,

Thank you for the pictures and the tape. How are you? How's Dad? I'm still very spastic, but am taking another Valium at suppertime. I must admit I'm not as depressed as I was. Dr. Tendy relieved my mind slightly, concerning my upcoming surgery.

I know you want to know about my Doctor's appointment. He took a look at me, and said I was a very difficult case. He gave me another appointment with a second specialist for February 15th. This doctor said that it would be a larger risk involved since I was older than he liked for this type of surgery. I feel like a rat in a maze, not knowing where to go or what to do. I like his honesty, and wish he would have told me more, but he wants a more knowledgeable doctor to tell me what might be impossible. I can't help but be nervous yet knowing God's behind me lets me walk through this smiling. The love from Him, and your love, makes my life happy and exciting. He knows what's good for everyone! The doctor is writing Grand Rapids for my last X-rays, from '74'.

If I remember right, Barb did go with me to that February 15th appointment. I was very apprehensive and longed for it to be over with.

3/20/79

Dear Mom and Dad,

Shaker, our new activity programmer, gave devotions last Friday night. The main idea was God never gives us anything we can't handle. I really thought about it over this past weekend, and if you read 1st Peter; verse 4 it states, "Yet if any man suffers as a Christian let him not be ashamed; but let him glorify God on his behalf." Shaker knows how to stir up my mind, and generate new concepts to dance within my awareness of life. I was happy to learn that I'm not "an impossible case" but still scared. I never wondered more about myself than in the past three months. I know Dad said, "Think it over. Don't rush into anything!" I thought about what I could do for ten long months, yet, the end justifies the means.

I had a bad curvature of the spine. In fact, when I was sitting in my chair, I could easily lay my head on my armrest. Dr. Westphal said that I needed two spinal fusions or I would end up flat on my back by my 40th birthday.

Dear Mom,

A reporter is coming out to interview me tomorrow, which might help my poetry get off the ground. I'm very excited because I'll be a featured story in our local newspaper.

Chris is coming tomorrow. We became great friends and he's going on the Nashville trip with me in May. I plan to buy some bib-overalls so I will look country, even if I hate their music.

Gary A., the reporter, came and did that interview on me. He wanted to put a collection of my poetry together and illustrate it with wonderful photographs that he took. He had a small shop, on Main Street in Coshocton, and I used to sit in his shop and shoot the bull with him. We became great friends, and he promised we would get a book together after he took care of some old business. I guess he never got that business completed, for we never worked on my book.

People used to kid me about going to his shop. They would remark, "Be careful of his dark room." Gary walked around many fairs with me, and we could talk about anything together, but I lost sight of him when he moved to Columbus. Life goes on!

5/28/79

Dear Mom and Dad,

How are you? I had a beautiful trip to Nashville and Gatlinburg. I love Gatlinburg, mainly because our hotel was just outside of the Smokies. We spent three days in each city. We went through Kentucky, and I saw real blue grass. Saturday, we went to Opreyland all day, which was extremely crowded, and I prayed I wouldn't run over anyone. By the time the day was over, all that I bumped into was a pole. We saw two shows. One was called "Showboat" which was performed on an actual showboat. People danced and sang songs of the south. That night, some of us had a pool party at our hotel. It was relaxing.

Sunday was busy also. We went to a museum and saw E. Presley's car. That afternoon, we went to the Grand Old Opera. I couldn't get over how large it is! Monday was a six-hour trip to Gatlinburg and the mountains. I rode a tramway up an eleven-hundred-foot high mountain. My mere words can't describe the beauty of it. I loved that part of God's creation. Tuesday, we went through Christus Gardens. That's a magnificent museum in which Christ is represented in life-like form. We went up in a Space Needle and shopped. Wednesday, we spent all day in the Smokies. We even went to an Indian reservation, in North Carolina. I thought of you when we were in the Carolinas.

Dear Mom,

I'm happy! I was glad I told you of my decision last night. The knowledge of Christ being with me, anywhere I go, helps. Dr. Westphal is one of my two main doctors. I will go in October 10th and be tested for four or five days and, if my body can take all the tests, then all systems go for this adventure. The first surgery will take place on the 15th, at 8:00 A.M. They will begin with my front by taking many of my organs out and placing a rod beside my spine. Somehow, they will place hooks next to the rod to tighten it. I will be in ICU for around six days after this surgery.

I will go back to my room until they feel I'm strong enough for the second rod to be inserted in my back to reinforce the first rod. They won't know whether they'll be able to fuse it until they are in my back. They can't tell by X-rays, but believe me, they know what they are doing!

After this, I'll be back in my room for seven days, waiting for my brace. It may be a week or two before I get my brace made. At this time, I will spend two weeks getting used to the brace before going back home to Echoing Hills. I hope to be in my chair within two months. I will wear this brace for nine months. It can only be taken off an hour a day to wash if any sores develop on me.

I'm thankful that I got the chance to attend Joseph's wedding. My brother looked husband, as Maria walked down the aisle, in that small country church. I enjoyed listening to Maria's friend serenade her from the balcony.

9/12/79

Dear Mom,

I love you! As the day gets closer, I find myself needing you more and more. Judges 16:26 states, "Samson said to the servant who held his hand, 'Put me where I can feel the pillars that support the temple, so that I may lean against them." I'm getting frightened and need you like Samson needed the pillars. I'm not afraid of the operation, for I know that this is in the hands of God.

I found out that the 15th is the day of my first one and the 25th will be my second one. Both will be at 8:00 A.M. I know it might seem foolish but I would feel better if you could be there. One of the ladies here said you might be able to stay with her parents. They live in Columbus. I guess this is a time in my life when you mean more than all the smiles I have here.

My eyes are tearful as I type this. I may call you over the weekend. I'm less than 139 pounds now with only four weeks to go. The less I weigh, the better the operations will turn out.

We're going to Holiday on Ice next Wednesday. That will be fun!

God bless.

9/17/79

Dear Mom,

I love you! You made me so happy when you said that you'll be there. I got some information on rooms for you and Dad, if you want to take them. The head nurse here called Children's Hospital, and they have eighteen rooms in Tinker Hall for parents of kids in this hospital. I better copy her note word for word.

Oh, she writes, "When parents come to the hospital, check with patient unit manager department, on third floor. No guarantee that they [meaning you] could get a room there. If not there, you'll be helped in finding accommodations." They said they put your name on a list to find a place. They also said that you wouldn't be more than ten minutes away from the hospital. You see, Tinker Hall is part of this hospital. They didn't give any idea on the cost.

As you can see, I'm getting shaky as the day nears. I'm planning on using all my typing things up to the eighth, as I won't be using them for a long time.

I can't put into words how much it means to me to have you near. God has blessed me with two beautiful parents

10/1/79

Dear Mom,

I need you! I cried today because I know Dad hates traveling, and you seem to do whatever he wants. I never needed you more than I do now! I love you so deeply, and if Dad doesn't want to make the trip, will you come alone?

I can do all things through Christ who strengthens me. He knows I'm human and that's what seems to be getting me down! He's right beside me so why must I crave to be near you, even if you have to come alone?

I went to Children's Hospital, in Columbus. The first of my surgeries was on the 10th of October 1979. This surgery was done on the front of my spine. You may wonder how the doctors reach and perform surgery on the front of the spine. Well they made an incision on my right side, moved my internal organs from the inside of my body to the outside, placed the rod in my spine, put my organs back inside and sewed me back up. This procedure took nine hours. My second surgery, for the back of my spine was on the 15th. This operation also took nine hours. You might say that they knew me inside out. I happened to be the oldest kid on the third floor yet, those five weeks were quite an adventure.

Carol, the head nurse, got the high honor of giving me two enemas the day before the anterior section of my trunk was opened. Believe me, this was an extremely moving experience. By the time it was over, Carol nicknamed me 'Brown Eyes'. At the nurse's station, they had a large black board that had that day surgeries written on it. Well, I talked Carol into writing GRAND OPENING under my name.

Dear Mom,

How are you? How's Dad? I was sidetracked by Shaker this morning, and ended up spending an hour talking with him. He almost called me a hermit, partly because I don't attend their Bible studies! I'm keeping too much to myself, or so he said. Ever since I came back from the hospital, I don't feel comfortable talking to many people around here. I don't tell Shaker that but that's how I feel. He said, we have to be involved in classes like cooking or music. We are narrow-minded if we don't take an active part in their groups. Mom, some residents can't even relax because of homework and Bible studies. Reverend Brown told me, before I even moved here, to keep busy and out of my room. Well, I know some residents who only come out of their room for meals.

Anyway, they're almost finished with the new section of the home. Once it's open, we will have the yellow living room for our typing room. Shaker said we could each have our own.

Here's a letter I found a few weeks ago. I didn't write Dad much, mainly because he stayed inside himself. I never really had a deep conversation with him yet, a few years after I moved to Echoing Hills, I wrote him a very honest letter.

3/4/80

Dear Dad,

How are you? I don't normally write you, which is my fault, but I need to tell you so much. I guess Mom told you of my poetry, and the chance of it being published. I'm finally doing something with my writing, and yet I'm frightened! I wanted to say, "Hey look Dad, I'm not just sitting around!" For so many years, I have sat in my room. People say I'm different since I came back from the hospital. Well, I am but they don't like me now. Mom taught me to accept people the way they are, so why can't they accept me.

People say that I'm a hermit, and am self-centered. I grew a lot over the winter, and not just in size! I'm speaking up more, and doing what I believe in, yet I'm getting in trouble more. God created everyone, and I'm just doing His will, but I feel so alone. What can I do?

I got my first rejection, from a magazine, in March of 1980. At first, I thought I failed my parents but then I recalled what I said in a Sunday school class once. It was not the right time, in God's plan, for me to be published then. How do you smile in the face of rejection?

Dear Mother,

    How are you? I really wish we didn't live so far apart. I miss you! Last night I took Debbie to a movie. The language was vulgar so we walked out of the cinema. A man saw us leave, so he gave Debbie a free pass that's good for any other movie. Actually, it's my pass, because I paid her way into the movie, but she took it and plans to give it to Shaker. Mom, how do you stand up for yourself?

    I sent away to another magazine yesterday. I don't want to be dead before I'm popular. I'm tired of asking for money from you.

5/2/80

Dear Mom and Dad,

I'm up to fourteen rejections. So far, I mailed forty letters to publishers and Kevin is now kidding me about the number of stamps that I'm using for all these letters.

I'm invited to lunch Tuesday, the 6th, at Children's Hospital. I know the food is bad yet I can't tell you how much the people mean to me.

I really worked hard on getting my poetry published. In my mind, that would show my parents that I am good for more than sitting on my butt. I recall sending two poems to over two hundred publishers around America and getting that many rejection slips back, with a cute little note saying, "You're to deep" or "You don't fit into our line of writing."

6/29/80

Dear Mom and Dad,

I'm going back to Dr. Westphal on the 17th. There's more pain in my lower back, than I like. He wants me X-rayed without the back brace to see if the rods are holding or not. If not, I'll have to do both operations over again. I am nervous about that prospect. I'll see another doctor about my foot, on the 11th. I know they will want me to wear a brace for that bone, but someday I pray to walk.

9/9/80

Dear Mom,

I'm tired today because I swam six laps of our pool yesterday. That seems to be the only way I can move freely. Next year I plan to swim in the Cerebral Palsy games.

We have a new program director by the name of Dan S. He's going to replace Mr. Kale on January 1st of next year. He seems to care, and is easy to talk to. Kevin, my counseling staff, and I talked with Dan for more than an hour today. The state's requiring more and more documentation on us, which pulls Kevin away frequently. He doesn't have time to talk much because he's doing five jobs now, besides planning his wedding in May.

That wedding is something I may never forget. It happened in mid May, in a Nazarene church in Coshocton. I never met Penny before their wedding day, yet you could tell their life was packed with love. Kevin was built, short and handsome, in a white suit, and Penny was plump and extremely sweet. Kevin was forever talking about her, but never described Penny's physical features. Anyway, the wedding was beyond beautiful. Their life together lasted six weeks, because she was hit, head on, by a semi. She was coming home from work, and one of her contacts fell out of her eye. I went to the funeral. Kevin was very brave through the whole ordeal, yet he joined the Peace Core eight months after her death. The memories were too much for him. I believe God never gives us more than we can bare, yet since we are all different, God gives us each our own assortment of adversities.

Dear Mom,

How are you? I've been sick since the first part of November. I moved my desk into the TV room in order to type. They are still working on the typing room, which is why I moved in here.

We are going Christmas shopping on December 6th, in Columbus. Carol's sister, Mary, might go around with me. The shopping center is only five minutes away from Carol's apartment.

How's Grammy? Please keep me informed of her health. I'm praying for her. We are having a farewell party for Mr. Kale on the 24th. He's moving on the 29th.

I recall the Christmas of 1980 all too well. Carol's family had invited me to their house for Christmas day. At Echoing Hills, when you could go home, to anyone's house, it was a triumph. You see, we had two kinds of residents. Those who went home on every holiday and those of us who couldn't for one reason or another.

Take Ralph, for example! Reverend Brown found him living in the basement of his mother's house. Ralph had Muscular Dystrophy, and his mother was ashamed of him so his early years were spent on the floor of her basement. By the time Reverend Brown found him, rats were dwelling in his hair and Ralph ate off the floor. His mouth was the only facility he could use, and man, he either praised you like a lover about to take you off into the sunset or cursed you until you thought you were in Hell! He was absolutely a lady's man. Much of his days were spent leaned up against four pillows, on his bed, watching TV or all the females passing his doorway. Every September he would stay awake all night for the Jerry Lewis telethon hoping someone would find a cure for MD.

Anyway, getting back to that frightful Christmas of 1980, Ralph was having trouble breathing. He went to his stepbrother's on Christmas Eve. Somehow he knew that he wouldn't come back to Echoing Hills. He never saw his 22nd birthday. Here's a letter that I wrote on New Year's Eve, after the shivering reality of forfeiting a friend.   Carol and I became close that summer. We went to the State Fair together to celebrate my coming out of my body brace.

11/29/80

Dear Mom,

How are you? I feel odd! I never cried when seventeen residents went home for Thanksgiving but today, when they came back, I bawled for about forty-five minutes. I'm not in the mood for Thanksgiving, probably because holidays were created for families. Echoing Hills had a big meal, and I pigged out, yet I wasn't in a festive spirit.

Kahlil Gibran, my favorite author, states it this way; "You may give them your love but not your thoughts. For they have their own thoughts. You may house their bodies but not their souls. For their soul dwell in the house of tomorrow, which you cannot visit, not even in your dreams. You may strive to be like them, but seek not to make them like you. For life goes not backwards nor tarries with yesterdays. You are the bows from which your children, as living arrows, are sent forth. The archer sees the mark upon the path of the infinite, and He bends you that His arrow may go swift and far."

I feel like an arrow lost in a bare field. Deloris, the staff who brought me to Grammy's house, never took the money that you sent me to pay her with. She's sick now and may not work for six weeks. Anyway, her family's poor and still doesn't have her last hospital bill paid off. Betty, her mother, is a staff here also. Could you possibly help them out?

12/31/80

Dear Mom,

How are you? Carol took me home for Christmas day and her family really made me feel welcomed. Each of them gave me a gift. Carol gave me a beautiful purse and some stationary. I ate a great home cooked Christmas dinner with a glass of wine. Her mother reminded me of you. On my way home, Carol told me that I did a lot of good for her parents. In fact, it was her mother who invited me in the first place. That really surprised Carol, because her Mom cries just by walking into a hospital. Her Dad didn't talk to me much, yet as the day went on, he seemed to be mellowing out.

After Carol drove me back to Echoing Hills, Georgia told me that Ralph passed away on Christmas morning. I cried! For awhile I was afraid to close my eyes yet, when I finally did, I saw God running right beside him in a heavenly baseball game. His step-Dad asked him three times if he was ready to go home. Ralph said yes, knowing in his mind that he would never go back to Echoing Hills. Some of us went to his viewing Monday and then Dick, his roommate, and the representative of the home went to his funeral Tuesday. It's sad to go past his room now. I loved him like a brother.

The administration wanted the residents to roll down to the multi purpose building for a church service. The bus wasn't going to run because of the four inches we got, last night. Since I didn't want to go outside, I typed. They don't believe I knew the Lord because I stayed back. Tommie was my second roommate, during this period of my life at Echoing Hills. She was a Quadriplegic, and was prone to infections. This was my first experience living with someone who uses a catheter. Tommie was still very sick, from yet another infection, and I didn't feel like going out into the cold anyway.

3/12/81

Dear Mom and Dad,

Tomorrow, I'm going to a branch of Ohio State University to see a counselor about starting college this fall. Dan S., our program director, is going with me. He's very interested in my writing, and like me, is sick of seeing me spending my life sitting on my butt. I have a talent and I'm going to use it!

Dear Mom,

I love you! God has blessed me with a happiness, I never thought I could have. Mom, I met a man named Richard in Maryland. I am very excited and glad to be alive! I wish you could meet him. Maybe you will someday. When this home gets me down, I just think of Richard and fly!

I'm starting to look for new homes now. Echoing Hills is taking too much of my freedom away from me, and I can't afford to lose what little I had.

I had a good time at John's wedding. The reception was beautiful, especially when John took Lena in his arms, and swirled her around the dance floor. They met in dance class.

Friday, I stayed up till midnight typing a term paper for Philosophy. I'm ashamed of my grade in that class, and feel that my best just isn't good enough. I'm working on a B. in my government class.

If memory serves me right, Richard was a veteran of the Vietnam War. Did you ever notice how you feel when another person pays you special attention. It's even a superior feeling when that person happens to be the opposite sex. You tend to see life as being beautiful no matter what might come along. I met Richard in Sandy Cove, Maryland at a Bible camp.

Richard thought it was love at first sight and kept telling me about all the things that we could do together. Like a foolish schoolgirl, I believed everything he told me. We planned to celebrate Thanksgiving together. He told me that he would make the ten-hour drive down from Delaware, and we would have a great holiday. I spent the Eve of Thanksgiving waiting for him. People began to think I wouldn't go to bed that night because I had already skipped supper and it was getting close to midnight.

"Did anyone call?" I rolled up to the nurse's station for the twelfth time. It started snowing around 8:00PM. and I was concerned.

The nurse shook her head. By this time, everyone knew what I wanted before I opened my mouth. "You better go to bed, It's late and we will wake you if he calls."

Ken and Pat were a third couple who got married June 27, 1983. They moved up to an apartment setting, which was built for wheelchairs. Ken died of a heart attack on May 4, 1991, but Pat had to move back to Echoing Hills because of health reasons.

The three married 'love birds' all had some common characteristics. For one, they all were very possessive of each other. Ken was always going in the bathroom while Pat took her bath. At one time, all three couples lived in the same hallway and when they fought, I heard about it! Only trouble is Barb and Jerry both had a speech impairment, which made it impossible to understand what they were fighting about!

We had many funny experiences, like the time Jerry and Barb ate supper next to me. All of a sudden, Jerry reached over and honked the horn on my wheelchair. He exclaimed, "Man, are you ever horny tonight!"

God does everything for a reason. In 1988 Don T. had very rough time breathing and ended up moving to the extensive care unit at the hospital. Sue spent three years riding the transit into town each morning, and then back out to the home again at night just to be with him. Sue moved into an apartment, in Coshocton, to be closer to Don. He wanted her to move to town to have easier access to him, yet I heard she sees him less now. She's having difficulty taking care of herself. I think the fact of being near him blinded her of all the responsibilities that go with living out on your own.

I realized that my first twenty-three years of life were extremely sheltered. I knew Mom was only trying to protect me but, in so many ways, her security is the basis for my confusion. No matter if I do have Cerebral Palsy, I do have the ability to love and be loved! I had my share of infatuations in my younger years, yet I couldn't turn to my own mother for advice. The mere thought of a man taking an interest in me was nons ensical.

This concept, about men, was shaken up when Jim came into my life! I dare not say too much, concerning relationships with the opposite sex, to Mom. Dad didn't care that much but Mom thought it was taboo. Jim was the shortest Texan I ever met. He was only 4'10" yet had a very compassionate heart. We would be the first ones in the dinning room, for meals, and the last to leave. We could talk about anything, and still had more to say at the next meal. I know residents could have behavior problems all around us yet, Jim and I would be so involved in our own conversation that we never heard anything.

January 9, 1991 was a night I will never forget! Jerry was typing on his autobiography when Pete B. and Randy B. went into that typing room to work on their computers. They had a bad habit of cursing whenever they got overly enthusiastic, or upset, about their work. Now, Jerry was raised with good Christian standards and got extremely hyper when these guys got into another swearing contest. One of the nurses, who really didn't understand any of us, came in to try to settle the affair. As normal, she made matters worse and Jerry went to his room madder than a wet hen! I lived in the room next to Jerry and Barb's. I must have woken up around 11:00 PM. because there was some kind of commotion in the hallway. The emergency squad was there. I learned later that Jerry died of an aneurysm in his neck. I was just getting to talk with him when God took him to paradise! Barb and Jerry were married seventeen years. Sometimes they fought, like any married couple, yet they had their passionate nights too. Barb was doing ok, the last time that I called.

On December 9, 1991, I only knew of two residents who I could actually hold down a meaningful conversation. Barb E. who lost her husband nine months ago tonight, and Sue D. who was my roommate before this nightmare came to life! My hallway was still in the section labeled I.C.F.M.R.D.D facility which would convert over to a nursing home facility by October of 1992. Sue did have a kidney transplant that past March so she was a good candidate for the first hallway to be converted to a nursing facility. We had three halls and mine was the next to convert. Sue and I made the VIPs write, and sign, a paper stating that we would be roommates again as soon as my hall is converted.

As I recall that frightening night, the nurses station at Echoing Hills received a call from the hospital, around 7:00 PM., saying that they had a kidney for Sue. She was one of forty residents who went to see a dress rehearsal at the Footlight Players Theater in Coshocton. Did you ever get so excited, yet so teary eyed all at once? Bob P rushed her back to pack an overnight bag. I watched as a staff threw what little Sue took into her travel bag. That moment had been what we were waiting on, for so many months, and now they had a possible donor. Sue went to dialysis every Tuesday, Thursday, and Saturday for a three and a half-hour treatment. She had to travel all the way to Zanesville for this treatment, which made her get up at 5:00 A.M. on those mornings. This would be rough on anyone so Sue had to take naps more than she wanted to. Sue was packed and going out of our driveway by 8:30 PM. I had an idea of what must go through the mind of a mother when her child is deathly ill.

The hospital called at 12:45 A.M. to report that they did Sue's blood work, and everything looked good for her transplant later that morning. The surgery would take around three hours and Sue was in great spirits. It's so awesome to know that God will never give us more than we can handle! It was March 22, when Sue came rolling in the door looking better than she ever had. This is one of God's magnificent miracles that could only happen with His loving hand. I always wonder how our Lord feels about major surgeries, like Sue's transplant. God gave doctors the beautiful talent of healing some, while others passed away to another life.

Sue was engaged. In fact, at one time, they had set a date for September 7, 1991, but then they had postponed their wedding when she found out she needed dialysis. I recall, around three weeks before they found a donor for Sue, Jim wrote to tell her that he was in love with someone else! She didn't really need that! Sue's an extremely emotional person. In fact, this was the second time we were roommates. The first time was a total nightmare! She would burst out in tears whenever I opened our bedroom door. If I looked at her the wrong way or didn't speak at certain times, she would erupt like a volcano! This can give a person a complex, after a while, so we had a room change.

12/17/81

Dear Mom,

How are you? We've around five inches of new snow already today, so I canceled my Doctor's appointment and rescheduled it for Spring break. If I have any problems before then, I am to give Dr. Westphal a call and get checked out. I was going this time because I was having pain in my hips and losing sleep. I kept reminding Mrs. Bailey about my restless nights yet she got her way by letting me wait till Spring break.

Oh Mom, I want to be my own person and I have a good mind to do it! Around Echoing Hills, the concept of caring for the individual person is rapidly vanishing. I want to express my needs more, but they always seem to get shot down. I have got to find another home before I lose sight of myself! Jim, the resident from Texas, knows of some homes down there, and he's going to give me the addresses of them. I even went over to Dan S. and got names of homes from him. I hate to deal with these people but he's the Director of Development and I knew he would have some ideas. Richard never called last Saturday. I was a fool to believe everything he said. Maybe you're right in saying that no one could ever want me for me.

Being unable to use a pen or pencil made life even a bigger challenge than you may think. I can't write checks or sign greeting cards, yet I am now a published poet and used to do some secretarial work for my Occupational Therapist and a few of the staff at Echoing Hills. People had nicknamed me the 'Unicorn Lady' down through the years. I started placing a rod in my mouth, which gives me more freedom, because I don't need help strapping a helmet on my head. People are glad I type with my mouth because I can't sing with the radio anymore.

I really wonder why God kept me in an institution for so long. Once upon a lifetime ago, I was sitting in my doorway watching staff go by, and wondering when I would use the bathroom or go to bed. One morning a few days ago, I listened to staff talk between them as one washed my private body parts as fast as they could. They were in a rush to get their work done so they could sit down and complain about how much work they had to do. Did I count? Did anyone ask me how my day was going or if I had someone special in my world? After all, I was just another resident in a nursing facility. This went on for sixteen years, eight months and thirteen days.

The state of Ohio was kind enough to pay for a counselor, someone to talk to me. There were eventually fifty-one residents at Echoing Hills; not many could be trusted, including the staff. Not many have that sincerity which the "good old gang" had so many years ago. A stranger is merely another human being striving to be accepted until that first initial "Hi!" Very few have that compassion which we felt before Echoing Hills became an institution for higher learning! A state funded rehabilitation center since 1985, when the government came in and transformed this home into a training facility! Reverend Brown needed more funding, in order to keep his central home opened and so goes the homey environment.

Well, if we were to receive funding from the state, we had to have two new requirements in order to live here. Let me explain these conditions which transformed my happy home into an instructional training center. I moved here assuming that Echoing Hills would be my home forever, if I chose it to be. The state insisted that the residents be actively involved in a structured life-style sixteen hours out of the day. These programs, as they call them, are daily living skills that teach a person such talents as washing their face, feeding themselves, and making sure they can balance a check book, among various other skills that you take for granted. For physically disabled people, even tying their own shoe can be quite a challenge!

And then we come to the second requirement, called zones. Zones were not as personal as programs and are similar to classes in school. We had reading, spelling, safety and cooking zones, just to name a few. We even had a leisure activity zone, which doesn't leave much time for ourselves. I gave up attending these activities because they were geared towards low functioning people. I needed to stimulate my mind and that "training facility" didn't do it anymore!

Chapter 5

Higher Education

"Now a touching things offered unto idols, we know that we all have knowledge. Knowledge puffeth up, but charity edifieth."
First Corinthians 8; 1

I will tell you about an excellent deception that lasted for a year and three weeks. I used to love the idea of attending college; I could work my brain as well as being with people who have the same intellect as I do.

It all began in 1980, when I started going to Ohio University in Zanesville. I was very fortunate to take this 45 minute drive, three days a week, with another resident by the name of Hiedi P. Now, the residents, nicknamed her 'mouth' which may give you some idea of how quiet my ride was? I mean to say, she knew about everything that anyone talked about!

We took this drive on the Coshocton Public Transit. After we used the hydraulic lift to get up into the bus, we had lock downs to secure our wheelchairs. If we were really fortunate, they might hold for half the trip. I knew when their van pulled up; we were in for an extra treat! We had to be manually pushed up two ramps that weren't fastened to the van. My wheels would turn which, at times, caused the ramps to slide. Talk about getting gray hair! Some rides to school were more exciting than a trip to an amusement park.

When we finally arrived at Ohio University, Phyllis T., the dean's secretary, would help us off with our coats and get our books for our first class. I thought something was peculiar, during that first year, Phyllis even assisted me in the restroom. I mean, how many deans would allow their secretary to wipe a student's butt?

Wheelchair people find it easy to carry a bag over their back of their chairs to keep the essentials of life in. By the third week of school, I felt I needed a U-haul! My first class was on the second floor with Dr. Arnold. Now this professor reminded me of old Tom Edison. He's extremely knowledgeable but, somehow, I can't visualize Dr. Arnold out in a field holding a kite. Philosophy was his class and so, for two and half-hours we would be lectured on great thinkers like Aristotle, Socrates and Einstein. Why, we even discussed Sigmoid Freud! Now, he was a demented, sex crazed, individual if I ever knew one. Once I got out of one of Arnold's classes, after hearing about so many different philosophies, I felt like rolling down the stairwell! All those concepts thrown at you at once would make anyone buggy!

I also had Dr. Jordan for Political Science. Now, this guy was a cool-cat! I cannot write so Dr. Jordan would give me my exams verbally. We would go out into the hallway and he would sit on the floor to ask me questions that were on the test. The students walking past would give us the strangest looks. I had Mr. Ware for my writing instructor. This is my specialty, for I have been a poet since I was nine years old. I got As and Bs in his class.

1/21/81

Dear Mom,

After Christmas break, my writing class started up again. I did not go because I have a bad cold. I called Mr. Ware up to get an idea for our next paper. He wanted a press release but, since I can't read newspaper print, he excused me from that assignment He also told me that I'm doing exceptionally well in other areas of my writing.

Take care.

College was excellent for my social life. One afternoon, I was rolling around the school's cafeteria be-bopping to the P.A. system's radio when my eyes caught sight of a totally handsome hunk of God's creation! Now, what was really unique to this setting was that he had a Bible opened in front of him. I recall his table was in the corner so I slowly rolled his way. Dave was his name and he was studying to be a biologist. We began talking and I found out that he was a true believer in God. We used to talk about everything from evolution verses creation to the memorization of each bone of a cat. Every week it seemed like he had a different animal to dissect for an upcoming exam. My Mom taught me that it's good to keep repeating, to someone, whatever it is that you want to memorize. This started to be a routine for us. We met in the lab once or twice a week. At times, this place became eerie with all the carcasses lying around and skeletons lurking in every corner. Dave and I sometimes met in the back of the school's library. We ate supper there on cold winter's nights. This was the start of my long career of breaking rules, which taught me what I could get away with and what it meant to be punished.

Let me tell you one thing, it's extremely hard to become your own advocate if you haven't been raised in the technique of defending your potential. I applied for a seat on the governor's counsel for physically disabled people. This is the type of work that I wanted to get into. It would also help me form a network of organizations, which may help me better myself. I really want to speak out for people who are, or will have the same difficulties that I am experiencing in my life. Being on the developmental Disability counsel would be a good step towards a brighter future for me. I wanted to major in graphic arts, if it was possible to do the work on my computer, and minor in business administration.

I really wanted to attend a Personal Care Attendant rally held on the State Capital. I thought this would be my big chance to display to society that the physically disabled are, in fact, a very important sector who only require slightly more help getting into the mainstream than the "normal" people of this world. Esther tried her best to get transportation that wouldn't cost me the world, but to no avail! The actual rally would only last an hour, and there was no guarantee that I could voice my opinion. Once I got there, I thought I failed. I even called Mom, two days before I was suppose to go, and teased her about bailing me out of jail if I caused too much of a disturbance. Can you imagine me in a paddy wagon? After all this excitement I was only disappointed, I was unable to get a ride to the rally. I thought to myself "Better luck next time!"

One experience took place, many years back, when numerous physically, as well as mentally challenged people require training in the various occupations that they want to pursue. Ms. Jones was a counselor for Vocational Rehabilitation, and I was on her caseload. Terry, and I became good friends, she was paralyzed and used a wheelchair. She drove a small sports car and owns a large, white fur, German shepherd. I really admired Terry and hoped to follow in her tire tracks once I get my own professional life in order. She recommended the purchasing of a computer before even attempting tackling the business world. Since I would be using it primarily for my daily living skills, Terry had to refer me to another division of Vocational Rehabilitation, which is called the Independent Living Program.

This bureau didn't have a permanent counselor at the time of my transition from Vocational Rehabilitation to the Independent Living Program. Ms. Karen Barnett was a temporary person until they hired another counselor for this department. Karen has dark hair and only one eye. She had a chauffeur, who impressed me to no end, and we had a great working relationship. If she couldn't meet with me in person, she would contact me by phone to update me on her latest endeavor in my quest for more independence. I recall our first face-to-face meeting. It was on April 11, 1990 and I did everything in my power to make her first impression of me a memorable one. I showed her my type-art and only my finest works of poetry. She loved them! I finally felt that I was going places with Karen. She set up an extensive computer evaluation on June 23, 1990, and I asked my best friend, Diana, to go with me.

This expedition started out at 9:00 A.M., and was a good three and a half-hour journey to St. Elizabeth's Medical Center in Dayton Ohio. Diana had the extreme pleasure of riding sideways in a public transit bus as she sat next to me. You never really lived until you travel somewhere sideways. Looking out the side window can make a stomach do crazy things! I learned to concentrate on the front window, even if it can give me a crook in my neck at times. I went shopping, for 'junk food', a week before hand. I bought everything from peanuts and cheese and crackers to miniature candy bars. I made sure, if we did get lost on this venture to the unknown; there was no way we would starve to death! I mean, even our bus driver wasn't sure of our destination. I remember offering the driver some crackers yet found that he had brought his own mini feast. Great minds think alike!

We made it to St. Elizabeth's at twenty till 1:00PM. Diana and I found the receptionist and signed in. At 1:00 PM. we were lead to a room that had wall-to-wall computers and various adaptations as well as equipment for physical and occupational therapy. I thought, "What are they planning to do with me? No wonder they said the whole evaluation will take three hours." Five women came into the room and told me what their expertise was. If you think about it, no one really knows everything about anything yet they love to think they do! There was a physical therapist, an occupational therapist, a computer specialist, a speech pathologist and a student occupational therapist. This panel was very comfortable to work with. Some three hours later, I felt sorry this evaluation was over and we said goodbye.

Well, it was mid-September before Karen got the results of my evaluation back. I recall the excited voice over the phone explaining the system suitable for my needs but then, it happened! They hired a full time counselor for the Independent Living Program. I received a letter on October 7, 1990 stating that Ms. Barnett had turned my case over to a Mr. Green.

He never did send me a formal letter, stating that he was now my counselor. I finally got apprehensive about what this guy was doing with my case, and I called him shortly after New Year's 1991. He didn't know what I was talking about. Green was used to working mostly with mentally retarded people and, like many who never really assisted people who are high functioning, his first impression wasn't too favorable. I asked him about my computer. He said that he couldn't do anything for me, that I had to go through Vocational Rehabilitation, which started a Ping-Pong ball game between Terry and Mr. Green. This blew my mind and so I called Terry. Terry assured me that she would talk to his supervisor, which she did, but to no avail! Mr. Green had to finish the job Karen had started.

Did you ever glance at the cover of a book and assume the text would read as lovely as the jacket? Nilah, one of my staff at Echoing Hills, went to the library to pick up a novel for me. Well, I require large print, which limits my selection of reading material because our local library doesn't carry a wide variety of this type of book. Nilah brought back a western that appeared to be a romantic love story about a woman trying to get her father's inheritance before her uncle did. She married a man and had to travel across America to keep up this business arrangement she had. The book was thick, which made me wonder how this author was going to hold my attention. It did have some sexual activity yet, when I really got into it, this novel dealt mainly with a prostitution ring and how a pimp got his 'ladies of the night'. I gave up reading it because it was getting extremely rough. You wouldn't think this novel would be like that just by looking at the cover.

Let me reflect upon my first face-to-face encounter with this pigeonholed person. On February 7, 1991, I met with Mr. Green and his supervisor at Echoing Hills. I invited Esther, who was my Q.M.R.P. at that time, to sit in on this meeting. I haven't figured out the purpose of his supervisor being there. He never spoke during our meeting, and acted as if he was bored. Mr. Green had the nerve to shuffle his papers while he asked me questions, and then looked up at Esther to inquire what I said. I finally learned the meaning of rude and obnoxious. About a month later, Esther got a call from Mr. Green who wanted to purchase a talking device for me. The speech pathologist from St. Elizabeth's must have written that I was eighty percent unintelligible where my speech is concerned. I do have impairment yet I am capable of being understood by most of the people who I come in contact with.

Mr. Green called me and apologized for his rude behavior three weeks after that first meeting. He also told me where he got this information concerning my speech being eighty percent unintelligible. The evaluation did state, although my speech can be understandable, I would benefit by using a talking device. I politely told Mr. Green that I'm not about to allow some organization to buy a Five thousand seven hundred dollar machine that I would not use in two hundred and forty-five years! My words might sound slurred, like some alcoholic who hasn't slept in twenty-four hours, yet my voice is something I have control over. I'm not letting some talking apparatus take over a portion of what little freedom I have! My mouth seems to get me into various kinds of trouble, yet I'm actually proud of my ability to speak up for myself!

I finally got my computer on May 26, 1991. I recall that experience as if it was just yesterday. Mr. Green came on the previous Wednesday, alone with the trainer who he had hired for me. John H. was his name and he was extremely tall. Anyway, both carried in four boxes of various shapes and sizes. When they got everything in our typing room, Green remembered they forgot the main brain of my computer. After waiting nine months, this was very disappointing. We talked and tried my equipment on Randy B.'s computer. Well, the upcoming weekend was Memorial weekend so I thought I wouldn't get the main part for another week. John thought he could move an appointment, which he already had on Memorial Day, and bring the rest of my computer. Monday came and all the residents were expected to go to the fish fry and parade that happened every Memorial Day. Well, I never got a phone call and so I thought I was in for another boring fish fry.

It was 10:30 A.M. when John came in our back door with a large square box. My dull day became the birth of Maurice, my computer's name. Well, John ended up staying for seven hours that day showing me things and explaining what he hoped to accomplish with me. He has over twenty-five years experience with computers, and he could operate one in his sleep. He had a Ph.D. and appeared to be above us all. As months went by, I became more and more frustrated with my spasms. My parents taught me to respect people with an enormous amount of knowledge. He would tell me to push a key that did one command but I ended up pushing another key that got me into a whole different function. After John left, at the end of a session, I would go outside and cry. I even hit a wall once! Mr. Green came down, to tell me that John was upset, but not at me. John's main goal was to find another way I can activate Maurice and this was frustrating him. John came by to fix something on my printer one afternoon, and when we finished repairing the printer, John sat back and asked me how I was doing. I hate questions like that! I tried not to think of my self, mainly because I didn't understand where I was going in my life. I finally told him about my spasms and about how I wanted to do everything right for him. We cried! We prayed and then talked some more. I could clearly see him as someone who was striving for the same things that I was.

Chapter 6

Faith

Now faith is the substance of things hoped for, the evidence of things not seen.

Hebrews 11:1

Mom raised all four of us in the Roman Catholic faith. Before I grew too big for Mom to carry up the church steps, the five of us would go to mass every Sunday morning. I recall times that I had spastic fits during mass. Mom would lovingly calm me down, or take me out of the main sanctuary, until I could relax. I never really figured out why Mom didn't take communion when that portion of mass came. She always asked Lynn to push me up to the altar. They would brace my shaking head while the priest would place a morsel of bread in my mouth. It was at this moment that I was most embarrassed at my inability to function as a "normal" person. I thought, God would never forgive me for what I couldn't help, but do during mass. Little did I realize that God allowed Satan to inflict my misunderstood physical limitation for a purpose! A nun called Mom up on a Monday morning, and told her to never send me to her catechism class again because I wiggled too much, interrupting her teachings. Mom knew I couldn't help shaking. I had already told Mom that there were seven and eight year old brats who screamed and ran all over the place like wild Indians on the warpath!

It wasn't until Dad's funeral that I figured out that Dad was a Presbyterian. He never went to mass with Mom, and the four of us, claiming that he had to stay home to cook Sunday dinner. When I got too heavy for Mom to carry up the church steps, Dad had to watch me every Sunday morning. Dad cooked enough food, on those Sunday mornings, to last us all week. When we sat down to one of his roast beef dinners, we could almost plan that our school lunches would be roast beef sandwiches for the next five or six lunches. If Dad cooked beef tongue, I would have a tongue sandwich for three days after. No one would swipe lunch boxes with me.

Since I didn't attend mass any longer, I never really understood why. Mom still made me say one hundred and fifty Hail Mary's every night. She bought me a gigantic rosary that I could hold on to yet I still managed to lose track of where I was. I have tried an assortment of denominational faiths, when I moved to Echoing Hills, and came to a strong conclusion not to lock the Lord Jesus Christ into a four walled box, where you go to pray to Him one morning a week! Through the years that I lived at that establishment, Christ revealed to me that He's everywhere, at all times and no one has any right to judge me for not attending any form of a church. I believe God is coming back for His bride, not His brides!)

As I was raised Catholic, I started going to Sacred Heart church in Coshocton. Echoing Hills provided a bus every Sunday to drop off residents at five denominational churches. After all the up and down motions you do, during a Catholic mass even before the priest enters the room, you tend to be too exhausted to really hear the Word of God! People were forever quietly slipping out before the end of mass to avoid the rush when he finally finished talking, which always seemed disrespectful.

When we had expanded to a 51-bed facility, we had two buses that transported each resident to their specific four walled box. I estimated that it took a good five hours to be loaded on the bus, unloaded at the proper church, and then waited another forty minutes for mass, or the service, to begin and finish. Following a mere fifteen-minute sermon, we reversed the process of loading up the residents at the doors of their individual faiths. I thought, by trying another religion, I could hear more of God's Word. Boy, was I wrong about that concept. After two years of this up and down routine, I finally gave a Methodist church a try.

Now, people didn't appear to do calisthenics at the Methodist church, yet every word you said during this service was written down in a small newspaper. Some of the residents, who went to this church, even went to sleep as soon as the singing ended and the main part of the service started. This was forever annoying me because I always seemed to sit beside a fellow resident by the name of Jack M. Jack was a nice guy. In fact, we once were an 'item' before I realized that he was slightly too old for me. He would start snoring as soon as the sermon began. I went to church in order to hear a good message, and when all the hymns were sung, Jack would catch 40 winks. I thought, if Mom ever caught me napping during mass, she would be sure that I went to bed an hour earlier next Saturday night!

I remember having to wait in the foyer until the bus came to take us home. This was where I met some bizarre people and there were times it got very embarrassing. There were instances when old ladies came up to me and patted my head as if I were some kind of dog.

"It's so nice of them to let you out for a while!" People would remark, as if I was in a state prison. I understand some walking people hardly ever come in contact with physically challenged individuals and so it's only natural that they didn't know how to react. Once, a friend of mine was chatting with me while I waited for the bus and a woman, around thirty-five years old, came up to my friend.

"Does she talk?" The woman looked at me as if my skin was green and I was stark naked! "How did she get this way? Poor little thing!"

Mary Anne looked at me in amazement. "I don't know. Why don't you ask her yourself?"

"How old are you?" She asked in a loud voice, as if I was deaf.

Mary Anne stood there flabbergasted by this pointless ignorance while the bus finally pulled up to the door of the church. "Thanks for stopping." She gazed at the woman in discouragement. "Pat, your bus is here. Let me help you with your coat."

"Hope to see you again." The woman rushed away as if she just remembered that her roast was still in the oven.

Now, this next church was extremely hypocritical in that they were making judgments on all other categories of four-walled-boxes! I got tired of "coat-rack Christians" which was how that church viewed all other faiths! Those were the kind of people who left God at the back of the church after Sunday morning service. When they went home, they'd start cursing until the following Sunday, when they wear a holier-than-thou face! This drove me crazy.

There was a period, in my life, where I thought we went to church only on Sunday morning to confess what we did on Saturday nights. For the longest time I truly believed that the whole "sexual experience" was an unforgivable sin. This woke me up to the fact that God isn't just within these four-walled-boxes where people go when they need "spiritual guidance." I stopped attending any denominational church for awhile.

Chris G. started working at Echoing Hills in 1982. It wasn't long before we became good friends, and we could discuss anything. We could turn to each other when we needed a shoulder. He invited me to an unique non-denominational fellowship in the small town of Martinsburg. It was one of those microscopic towns that if you blink as you drove through, you might miss the one and only stop light. This gathering of twenty met in an old garage-type building that was the town's body repair shop. Community Christian Fellowship was the name of that tiny group of believers and Bob [Moose] Peltry was their preacher.

Bob was nicknamed Moose, because he was a tall man and looked like a team member of the New York Giants! Each Sunday, Bob had to set up a card table for his pulpit as well as folding chairs for people to sit on. He made a small wooden pedestal to hold his Bible and every week he would walk into the garage with this pedestal under his arm as if it was some sort of a football. I had to laugh each time I saw this because you hardly ever see a preacher who carries his own pulpit!

C.C.F. was where I first felt free to reveal, to this world, my relationship with the Lord Christ Jesus. We sang, danced and clapped for the King of kings! Some spoke in tongues! This frightened me at first, but then I realized that this is biblical.

In 1 Cor.12:10 God states, "To another the working of miracles; to another prophecy; to another discerning of spirits; to another diverse kinds of tongues; to another the interpretation of tongues;" I also gained knowledge about prophecy and how awesome God really is!

We spent around a year in that building. I recall celebrating New Year's eve of 1983 there. It was my first New Years eve party away from Echoing Hills (and I thought their parties were boring). I was extremely surprised to greet 1984, in total silence. New Year's eve only comes once a year. When I think of celebrating the old year out, I picture noisemakers, horns blowing and people shouting praise the Lord! Well, midnight came, and you could hear a pin drop!

Please don't misunderstand me, I'm a firm believer of praying, yet here's a time for rejoicing! Psalms 150:1 states, "Praise ye the Lord. Praise God in His sanctuary; praise Him in the firmament of He power." The power of a simple prayer is magnificent, yet I was ready to celebrate at the stroke of midnight. Oh well, a friend of mine always tells me that, at the stroke of midnight, the cows get down on all four knees and pray to God for a good new year! If they can do it, we best be doing it too.

The owner of this garage heard an ugly rumor that we were some kind of satanic cult and ordered us out of that building. Bob located a small, empty church out on State Route 97. It was white with a bright red door and four steps. This was a time when my faith has really put to the test. Each week, Chris, and three other men, pulled me up those three long cement slabs. The trust of God never fails!

It was here that I met Thorny, Julie K, and their children. They would take me home, every so often, to give me a break from my institutional environment, as well as to give me some home cooking. Julie had blond hair and buckteeth. She reminded me of a two-legged beaver with braces. Thorny was pleasingly plump and very good at preaching the Word of God. In fact, this family of four broke away from C.C.F. and started their own nondenominational church, called Christian Gathering. Thorny had been working at a glass factory before it closed because of financial reasons. If I recall, he found work in a prison camp for teenagers.

Isaiah.61: 1 states, "The Spirit of the Lord God is upon me; because the Lord hath anointed me to preach good tidings unto the meek; he hath sent me to bind up the brokenhearted, to proclaim liberty to the captives, and the opening of the prison to them that are bound."

C.C.F. was when I first remember being a cupid. Cupid is a kinder term than 'being used', yet it took me a long while to realize that, many of my encounters, are exactly those. I'm being used! One Sunday morning, a very lovely lady came up and sat next to me. We started to talk and I found out her name was Pam. She had her eyes on a man named Mike, who played the trumpet for our church. Pam wanted to get acquainted with this blue eyed wonder and needed some ideas on how this could be done. Well, I already was a good friend with him so, when he glanced over at me, I faked a spasm and dropped my hymnal. Pam began to pick it up for me but, like the gentleman Mike is, he rushed to my side to help Pam pick the book up. They started to talk and, they were married the following year. He became a doctor and they had three beautiful baby girls.

In Hebrews 10; 22 Christ proclaims, "Let us draw near with a true heart in full assurance of faith, having our hearts sprinkled from an evil conscience, and our bodies washed with pure water." C.C.F. was where I had the awesome experience of being baptized a second time. For me, this is an outward expression of an inward act! I had already acknowledged my personal relationship with Christ, yet others were hesitant to accept my word for it. It's like having to prove to society that you truly love someone. I always wondered why two souls had to show to others that their love for one another is real. No one can actually view authentic love between two people!

First Corinthians 3; 16 reminds us that, "Know ye not that ye are the temple of God, that the Spirit of God dwelleth in you?" I recall C.C.F. finally purchased an old van and built a ramp for wheelchairs to drive up into. Three other residents started attending this non-traditional church with me. This lasted for approximately two years. Our congregation grew until we had standing room only for Sunday morning service. Bob finally got tired of paying rent for the usage of that little white church, so he bought a section of land out on SR 229.

We built our own "house of God", which meant no more rent or getting kicked out for being known as a cult! Chris G. sang more and more, until he eventually quit his work as an orderly at Echoing Hills, to go on tour with a Christian singing group. I believe, nowadays, he's working on a cruise ship that travels around the world.

A few months after Chris stopped coming to C.C.F., the van started breaking down. Bob became extremely involved with the upkeep of his church so, when the van ultimately needed a major overhaul, my church family voted to carpet the sanctuary instead of repairing the van. I always wondered which was more important, the appearance of a four walled building or four souls. I stopped going there in 1986.

I stayed home for about a year and a half. By now, the concept of a church family was turning me off. One afternoon, I rolled into our TV room and turned on TV when, all of a sudden, Julie K. came into the room. It was a Wednesday in mid-January and they had Bible study at 6:30 PM. that night. Their small group of eight or ten met in a country church only five miles away from Echoing Hills.

New Guilford is one of those dinky towns that, if you yawn while driving through it, you may miss it. They held their services in the Methodist church, which just happened to be the only church in New Guilford. I rode past this building many times on the way to Columbus. I was very interested in seeing the inside of this miniature mansion of God so I took up Julie's invitation to come hear Thorny preach.

Acts 10;42 proclaims, "And he commanded us to preach unto the people, and to testify that it is he which was ordained of God to be the Judge of quick and dead." On the way to Thorny's Bible study, she refreshed my memory as to why Thorny broke away from C.C.F. She said that Bob didn't really appreciate Thorny getting into his territory of preaching. Thorny felt that this was a calling from God and so detached himself, as well as his family, from this sort of thinking.

If you are a genuine believer in the Lord Jesus Christ, you have an obligation to spread the Word of God to any soul who you come in contact with! Julie said that they call themselves "Christian Gathering" and meet on Sunday and Wednesday evenings. This congregation mainly consisted of farmer's wives. Thorny had his job cut out for him because their husbands worked late in the fields, yet expected each wife to be home to have supper on the table when they got home. Thorny tried very hard to have a moving message yet be done by 8:00 PM. Jr. was the man who led the singing and, like CCF, we danced and some talked in tongues while others interpreted.

At times, Jr. selected some of the gathering to lead Bible study. This gave a few of us a chance to speak about Christ in our own unique style. I once had the privilege of giving a Bible study on the theme of God's love. This was a very nervous night for me. Having speech impairment creates awareness in me to make each word I speak clear and precise. I have my own form of an accent. Many people find it uncomfortable to ask me to repeat my words, if they don't understand me, so I really pray to God that they get something out of my Bible study.

I recall my topic that night, was love and acceptance of one another. I remember I had a number of scriptures to refer to on loving. Julie introduced me to a strong, young guy by the name of Herbbie Y. His family is Amish and frowned on him when he discovered Jesus Christ as his personal savior.

In Revelation 22;13 God exclaims, "I am the Alpha and O'me-ga, the beginning and the end, the first and the last." He goes on to state that, "Blessed are they that do his commandments, that they may have right to the tree of life and may enter in through the gates Into the city." Now, if this man created each soul on earth as well as counting each hair on every head, don't you think he should be worshipped and adored? Oh, how awesome our God is!

Julie knew Herbbie could lift me up, like a groom does with his bride on their threshold, and position me in the car seat easier than she could. Herbbie picked me up twice a week. Wednesday evenings, for Bible study, and Sunday evenings for our weekly church service. At times, this was very embarrassing for I enjoy wearing skirts and dresses. My Mom would have a royal conniption if she knew I had a man lift me twice a week while I had some sort of skirt on! There were times when I thought he pinched my butt yet I couldn't prove it.

Then, Herbbie met, and dated, a woman by the name of Jeannie. She would come with Herbbie when he picked me up and dropped me off after evening service. Jeannie was a divorced woman and had a little girl by the name of Christi. She's a very sweet girl and I felt sorry for her, because every other weekend Jeannie's ex-husband would take Christi for Saturday and half of Sunday. If that girl was me, I would feel like a volleyball!

If that wasn't enough confusion, seven months into Herbbie and Jeannie's relationship, they became engaged. Now, Christi started calling

Herbbie daddy, as well as telling Jeannie what her real daddy got her every other weekend.

I had to take my manual wheelchair to this church because of the steps, just like C.C.F. Anyone who understands me knows that I hate being immobile! This meant that, once Herbbie parked me beside a pew, I stayed there until it was time to go home. This was OK at first because Julie would sit next to me and talk. Then, the novelty wore off. Julie wanted other people to get to know me so she began to sit away from me. Julie's idea didn't work. No one but a lady by the name of Beth came over she talked, laughed, and held my Bible for me. Beth was pregnant, at that time, so she didn't come to church every week. Her family drove two hours each time they came to church and, for a seven-month pregnant woman, the trip got to be too much for her.

I enjoy chitchatting like any other person. I really believe in building others up and not discussing the negative aspects of people. Since Beth hardly came anymore, few people came over to talk. They each had their own small circles that I never seemed to fit into. There were times when I thought I had forgotten my deodorant! After the service, people would gather to talk, or gossip, but they were all on the opposite side of the church. I was really wondering why I was even there.

In Psalms.71: 23-24 David states, "My lips shall greatly rejoice when I sing unto thee; and my soul, which thou hast redeemed. My tongue also shall talk of thy righteousness all the day long; for they are confounded for they are brought unto shame that seek my hurt." I needed more out of life than sitting there looking at others living.

I decided to try the Nazarene church in town. Yes, back to the bus routine. This concept made Christian Gathering uptight. If we truly are the body of Christ, it's good to get different viewpoints on God's Word to gain a deeper knowledge of this man called Jesus Christ. Thorny and his family were about to move to Africa to share the Word of God, yet I got frowned upon for attending another church!

It was the spring of 1988 when I started up a relationship with a man named Bob R. He worked in our central office that is just across our driveway. Echoing Hills is a large corporation now. When I first moved to Echoing Hills, this was the only facility they owned. At present, they operate several homes that are scattered around this state.

Bob worked on pay roll and billing for all the homes. He also sorted the house' mail. This is how we met. I would roll over to central office and get the resident's mail or, if 'things' became too hairy over here, I would simply roll over just to get away for a short while. Bob had red hair and always wore purple ties. I teased him about the color purple, and soon we became good friends. We started talking, as he sorted the mail, and expressing viewpoints on various subjects that were the topic of the day. We got to discuss "Christian Gathering" once when he reminded me that the residents of New Guilford were spreading rumors that "Christian Gathering" was some kind of a cult.

All these months, I wondered why this congregation hadn't grown over twenty people. It did seem as though they were keeping too much to themselves, as well as Thorny asking for more and more money for his family's move to Africa. This made me question the meaning of "A calling from God." If it were an authentic calling from our Lord, wouldn't it stand to reason that He would provide the way? I mean, God helps those who help themselves, yet many of the farmwomen didn't even have good housing conditions but he still asked for monthly donations.

I truly believe that God created each soul on this earth, to glorify Him. From reverends to taxidermists, atheists to car salesmen. Each is born with a mission in this life that no one else can accomplish! Everyone has a faith in someone or something. I don't believe in all those assorted denominations that think they are the only faith who will make it to Heaven! We are all striving to be accepted, and loved, as well as sharing the love deep within our souls!

It happened shortly after Dad's death. People at Christian Gathering gave me the impression that his dying never really mattered since Dad didn't actually claim Jesus Christ as his personal savior. My Mom told me that, during his final hours on this earth, Dad had a minister by his side. I loved him and always will. This was why I never went back to Christian Gathering. No human being has the right to condemn any other being to Hell. That's God's job!

Matthew 7; 1-2 states, "Judge not, that ye be not judged. For with what judgment ye judge, ye shall be judged; and with what measure ye mete, it shall be measured to you again." People are unique! They fear anything that boggles their mind. Larry A. knew I was moving to Toledo, and so he called his pastor friend Larry E. at Grace church up in Toledo. I moved to Plainsville Care Center on December 16, 1994, temporarily, and Pastor Larry E. came over the Thursday before Christmas. He brought me a care package of three kinds of popcorn, some cookies [which I gave to the nurse's station] some fudge and a book called "The Message". It's the New Testament in today's language. I was having problems with Maurice; my computer and Larry asked a deacon, by the name of Net, to come look at it. He is very knowledgeable about computers and it wasn't long before Maurice was back in great working order.

Janet is one of my best friends from Grace church. She came by one Sunday afternoon in January. Janet and her husband, Randy, wanted to take me to church on Sunday mornings. Pastor Larry found out that many of his members didn't know how to befriend someone with a physical disability, so he asked Randy to ask me to write a paper on Cerebral Palsy. Here is that essay...

"Will the circle be Unbroken"

Gen. 1:26 " And God said, Let us make man in our image, after our likeness, and let them have dominion over the fish of the sea, and over the fowl of the air, and over the cattle, and over all the earth, and over every creeping thing that creepeth upon the earth." Yet, God never specified what is "His image" and what is not. I believe that we are in His image for nine months and then the cord is cut! Satan has a field day with all of us. Some hide their disabilities well and others wear glasses or hearing staffs. Still others have visible challenges that this society has labeled disabled.

"Cerebral Palsy: paralysis caused by brain damage prior or during delivery, and marked by a lack of muscular coordination, spasms, and difficulties in speech." so a medical dictionary explains.

Job 1:8-12 states, "And the Lord said unto Satan, Hast thou considered my servant Job, that there is none like him in the earth, a perfect and upright man, one that fears God, and turns away from evil. Then Satan answered the Lord, and said "Does Job fear God for nothing? Hast thou not made a hedge about him, and about his house, and about all that he hath on every side, thou has blessed the work of his hands, and his substance is increased in the land. But put forth thine hand now, and touch all that he hath, and he will curse thee to thy face. And the Lord said unto Satan, Behold, all that he hath is in thy power: only upon himself put not forth thine hand. So Satan went forth from the presence of the Lord." I'm not saying that I am righteous than any other person! What I am saying is that I'm just like you. I'm a sinner and have mortal thoughts! We all fear the unknown, yet, how does the unknown get to be reality? There's so much about my own physical disability that I don't understand and, as years go past, I find that my inability to achieve many activities intensifies!

When I was young, I would strive to be as 'normal' as the people around me were. You must remember when you were growing up; you studied others and tried to imitate them. For years you modeled yourself after someone you thought 'had it all together' yet, somehow, you failed. That's what I did for so many years.

Romans 5:3-5 "And not only this, but we also exult in our tribulations, knowing that tribulation brings about perseverance, and perseverance proven character; and proven character, hope; and hope does not disappoint, because the love of God has been poured out within our hearts through the Holy Spirit who was given to us." In my life-style, I know the saving grace of God is what gives me the endurance to keep going. Everything on earth has some risk to it! From moving into your first house to befriending someone that's different than you yet has the same desires and expectations as you. When Christ walked this earth I'm sure He didn't hesitate to relate to people who weren't in the "norm."

In conclusion, we are each a valuable link to the infinite man called Jesus Christ. It's a great challenge to meet new and different people every day. He is our only way to eternal salvation! If you reserve your soul for people of your own kind, how will the circle of Christ expand to the far corners of this world?

Chapter 7

Camaraderie

"Let every soul be subject unto the higher powers. For there is no power but of God; the powers that be are ordained of God."

Romans 1:3 R

Getting down to the subject of a good conversation among friends, all but two of the 'old gang' have gotten married and moved away, or died!

When Dad passed away, I really needed to talk. I was tired of the home's counselor, her name was Pam, and started asking around for names of different ones. Pam seemed to get off the track and was interrupted by staff members. Teresa M., who was a staff at Echoing Hills, gave me the name of a counselor in town who's not related to the home in any way. That concept totally blows my mind! I mean, having new thoughts on old situations seems to brighten my view of myself! Echoing Hills didn't really enjoy the thought of not knowing my every concern but I value the private matters of my heart!

Pam and I might say an occasional 'hi' in passing nowadays but that's all. If Gary W. was the sort of professional who strictly 'went by the book', then I would had never made that June 4, 1990 appointment. My first impression of him was a total slob! I guess we all tend to stigmatize others even before we get to know them. Gary's a professional, and all I had visualized was a stuffed shirt in a black three-piece suit. You know the kind of people who usually make you feel as if you should pay them just to look at you!

Gary wore a motorcycle jacket and reminded me of some sort of a hoodlum just getting back from a caper. His office had a sandbox in a corner and a large picture window that overlooked a busy intersection of downtown Main Street. It seemed to be a lifetime of hour-long sessions and yet I got an odd feeling that these talks couldn't last forever.

Spans of moments in which I could cry and not be scolded for acting like a four-year-old in search of a hug! Many were screaming fits when I finally faced the bitter reality of a obstacle of life. Then, it started! I began hearing gentle hints of terminating my case until I finally didn't go back after April 24, 1991. That was exactly one year from the day Dad died! I have received a few letters from Gary since then. I recall a note that stated that I didn't really know the definition of terminate.

This letter came to me just after I came home from Ken P.'s funeral! I never went back to that office with a sandbox in it. Everyone needs someone. I have an intrinsic desire to be needed, and know that whatever happens in life, you could turn to some special person for comfort! Society teaches us that it's a sign of weakness to require staff, yet it helped me to know that I could talk to someone. I learned that I am physically and mentally unique, as well as gifted.

As years go by, I notice more and more people flowing with the crowd. We have others that go out of their way to be different. Cindy Lauper is extremely weird yet, when you think about it, she can leave a lasting impression. Imagine painting your hair bright blue and singing as if you were gasping for each breath you took. I admire people who are unique. Many think that, if you dare to be different, others won't accept you.

The other night I had my first passionate dream since my Dad's death. I woke up feeling extremely guilty because, at the time of Dad's passing, I made a vow to God that I wouldn't get romantically involved with anyone. I didn't feel that my soul could stand grieving over the loss of another male figure in my life. Through out my younger years, Mom warned me that no man could really love me! After all, I can't even feed myself or handle my own physical care. How was I ever about to imagine having a sexual experience with any man. You must consider that Mom said all this in a period when Dad was highly frustrated with his own life, and gave Mom Hell for three weeks at a time!

Most women my age have been married at least once, experienced sex, and maybe even breast-fed their children. Some man has claimed they needed her, slept with her, created a sense of security in her that each human on earth requires. Someone once said, "No man is an island!"

I'm no different, yet in this society, we must look and act like Madonna to gain this certainty that someone cares! Day after day, I hear my staff discussing who they were with the night before. How soft his lips were, and how gentle his touch was. Yet they would have another lover in two weeks or so! For the life of me, I cannot understand the concept of modern day love. Are they seeking perfection?

Frustration grows when we fight to understand something and fail! It seems to me that that's what life is, a series of experiences which we face each day, either accepting as a challenge, or rejecting as a negative aspect of life! In all reality, I couldn't handle sexual intercourse because of my muscular spasms yet this doesn't mean that a warm and tender man cannot hold me someday. There are nights when this prayer seems so far away yet God knows my heart! There were many lovers but they never lasted.

It's bizarre, how many bittersweet relationships I had over the years that I've lived at Echoing Hills. Many ended abruptly, by the power of death, yet numerous others still flicker in and out of my life as if God is reassuring me that I'm all of a woman! Take Valentine's day of 1985, for instance, if Scott had not agreed to accompany me, it would have been very boring.

We had an annual Valentine's banquet, and I got so tired of attending these affairs unaccompanied! What does one do alone at these functions, but stare at her plate and try to guess what the main course was. Three weeks before our banquet, I called one of our former orderlies whose name was Scott E. He went to work at the local town's newspaper. His back had gotten worse, plus he didn't see eye-to-eye with the administration of Echoing Hills. "Another one bites the dust," I always say whenever a good employee finally sees the light!

Echoing Hills was a very missionary oriented home. They felt that we should write inmates of prisons to share the Word of God and I got involved with a man named John Wasson. Scott was a great photographer. I hired him once when I was having an affair with a sex maniac of a pen pal. He was on death row down in Texas. John wanted to see whom he was writing, so Scott and I went into the home's chapel where he took at least sixty poses. Some were very interesting. My next letter from John asked for more pictures of me, but he wanted more of my female parts than I felt comfortable in revealing to him! I showed my leg, up to my thigh, but was embarrassed at the thought of exposing anything more! You may wonder why I kept in contact with a perverted sex-maniac.

Every woman likes to think someone loves her and I'm no exception. John's letters began to be very explicit and vulgar, dealing with only the sexual experience and what we would do in bed! I finally stopped writing

John. After four months, I sent him a Christmas card. He replied with a questionnaire type of a letter asking if I got married and if my husband could fulfill all my desires, like he did. I wrote my first "Dear John" letter and ended our pen-pal relationship!

Scott and I could talk as lovers, as two souls searching for that one magnificent fantasy that only leads to ecstasy! Whenever he caught me in one of my not-so-sure-who-I-am moods, he would come down to my level and whisper in my ear, "We are the two smartest people in this whole darn home!" Why must all the good people leave?

The night is when I think is the best period of the day to write of passionate lovers, who expressed their infatuation for me and then walked [or rolled] away! I recall a resident by the name of. Todd also has Cerebral Palsy, and is more spastic than I am. He isn't able to talk understandably, so he has to use an alphabet board, and hates restrictions just like I do. Todd thought he loved me, so he asked me to go steady, and bought me everything from thirteen roses, balloons and a pizza to a red and black dress for a conference that we ended up attending 'together'. At first, I thought this relationship was Heaven sent, but I soon felt as if he owned me. When I went anywhere, Todd always asked where, and who I was going to see. He wanted to know what time I would be back, and even what I would talk about while I was out. Every night we would roll back to my room and try to do what lovers do. We held each other, and tried to kiss. He didn't like my glasses, so I would race him back to my room and manage to wiggle my glasses off. Then, Todd would come in, would slam the door behind him and get his chair as close to mine as possible. We kissed and he managed to get one of his spastic arms under my loose nightgown. He felt what men crave for, and I really thought he would care more if I gave him what he wanted. Boy, was I ever wrong! This activity became something Todd expected of me every night. The activity in my bedroom became a kind of a ritual that made him satisfied, but it made me start to feel like a used woman-of-the-night.

I finally ended this relationship by writing him a letter. I was still grieving the death of my Dad, and all Todd could do was compare the loss of a football game to the death of a human being. He got my note and hurried to my room. Slamming my door behind him, he cursed me out and told me that I didn't mean what I wrote! I hate being called a liar. I rolled out of my room, thanks to a staff who opened the door after I screamed. "He won't let me out!" Tears rushed down my face as I rolled outside and cried some more.

Did you ever notice how a wheelchair degrades the person using it? I came to the conclusion that it must have been designed by a man, because it is highly belittling. After all, "The eyes are the windows to one's soul." At one time we had an orderly working here by the name of Philip B. I recall the time I finally 'broke the ice' and entered his world by complimenting him on how 'cute' his derriere is. In my world, all one comes in contact with are butts and belt buckles. We were comparing the various sizes of buttocks that work here. It's ridiculous, what people find to discuss at the dinner table.

Philip's a short guy with black hair and an unique way of walking. He was rolling our trash bin, which looks like a mailbox with casters on it, around the ten dinning tables that we had.

Chuck was helping to clear off the lunch table when he ventured to ask me why I hadn't opened the door to a new relationship with Phillip.

A good friend of mine by the name of Chuck overheard the conversation at my table.

"I don't know. He has a cute derriere!" I remarked, as I sipped the last of my coffee.

Chuck glanced over at Phillip. "You want some help?" I felt my face turning slightly red. "I dare you!"

Chuck and I had known each other since 1986 and he knew I take any dares put before me.

"Hey you, over there! I initiate many of the new staff around here, and the members of my table consider you to have the best looking derriere in the dinning room today!"

Phillip didn't understand my lingo at first, so Chuck echoed my words to him. He smiled. From then on he began to see me as the woman that I really am! He started to kid me about my spastic fits, and made me see the beauty of a shaky limb. We started finding situations in which we could talk, such as meal times or he'd invite me out on his fifteen-minute breaks.

One extremely embarrassing experience happened at snack time one evening. He was pouring our drinks when I rolled up behind him and patted him on his butt. At first, he seemed not to notice, so I brought the subject up.

"Hey, how did you like my fake spasm?" I asked with a smile.

"You better be careful! You could turn me on with your orgasms!" He exclaimed with a sheepishly grin. This was a time when my speech impairment caused a hilariously foolish moment when I felt like crawling under a rock and never showing my face again.

"What do you mean? I said that I faked a spasm. What did you think I said?" I inquired curiously.

"I thought you said orgasm?" He brought some red drink over to my table.

I looked up at him. "By the way, what's an orgasm?" I was as serious as the day I was born.

"You mean, you don't really know?" His face was getting as red as the drink he poured. I had unintentionally embarrassed him.

"I'm not dumb, please don't misunderstand me. I simply am not educated in matters concerning sexual acts. My younger years were too sheltered! Some say that I'm very naïve," I exclaimed, trying to prove to myself that I did know something.

Phillip walked back up the hall, so I made small talk with the staff who was feeding me. Five minutes later, he came back carrying my large type dictionary. He opened it to the Os. He pointed to the definition. "Here, read this." I felt myself wanting to crawl under the table.

Philip started nursing school in September in 1990. This was a one-year program and he went down to working part time during that year. We still had opportunities to talk, yet it was not as often. He graduated, with flying colors, that fall. Phillip started looking for a nursing position at Echoing Hills. His first meeting, with our illustrious administration, seemed favorable, so he passed up four better paying jobs and kept on working as an orderly did. They said they needed him on the floor for a few more weeks. This few weeks turned into a month. Phillip got called back into the celebrated administration's office, and was told they weren't hiring any more nurses. He was slightly more than upset and quit on November 3rd of that year.

February 3, 1991, will be a memorable afternoon for a long while. It was a beautiful spring-like day and I decided to take a roll [I never walk] up to our corner store. I guess I needed to prove to myself, as well as a fellow resident, that I could make it up the hill right before you drive onto long and twisted lane which led to Echoing Hills. State Route 541 is the highway just before turning on County Road 79. Now that was the longest driveway I have ever seen for a home. I talked one of our newest staff into walking up with me. Holly was her name and she needed counseling on her latest flame. I found I do make an excellent ear for friends and lovers.

The Post, as we used to call the corner store, reminds me of something out of a scene of Gunsmoke. A cowboy would stop to water his horse, shoot a little pool and then ride off into the sunset with a woman on his mind. Only problem with this picture is that society has modernized this site by putting in a concrete slab with two gas pumps for the convenience of modern day transportation. Anyway, the Post carries everything from candy and pop to over priced necessities of life! I like their pizza subs, and this was our mission, or so I thought. All the way up, I tried to discourage this romance, knowing that Scott R. had a reputation for blowing up a woman's self-image until he had her where he wanted her. Then, the novelty wears off! A new woman would comes to work here and he'd treat Holly like an old pair of shoes.

When we finally arrived, he just happened to pull up in his bright red truck. He had on a T-shirt and a pair of shorts. Holly ordered my hot pepper cheese pizza sub, and found out that we had a 20-minute wait. It's odd, how circumstances happen to take place at just the right time. Another resident just incidentally called the store and asked for that particular orderly.

"How long will you two be here?" He looked at Holly. "Pete wants a sub and they don't deliver today."

"We have a 20 minute wait," Holly answered excitedly.

"Would you mind taking a sub back to Pete? I'll wait around with you so you don't get bored." He turned to me.

"I'm in no hurry to get back to that nightmare!" I remarked. "It's a beautiful day out! Let's wait outside by the picnic table?"

"I just have to be home by 8:00 for a birthday party," Holly mentioned, as she pushed me across the gravel. The ground was extremely soft, and it felt that my electric wheelchair could have sunk deep into the grass if he wasn't with us.

They talked, as Holly held up my Pepsi so that I could drink it. Once again, feeling like a third wheel, I looked around to see the beginning signs of spring. Nervously, they talked about work, and what they might do on their next day off. Then, he went in and brought the subs out. After putting them in my backpack, he aimed me out of the gravel and onto the pavement. We decided to go home, so I started down the hill. I had no idea that Holly wasn't behind me, holding me back, until I started going into the ditch. My head hit a drainpipe and I ended up with six stitches next to my left eye. That night, I hardly slept. I felt used and abused from an evening in the emergency room. I felt I had lost something of myself, as people came into my bedroom every half-hour to see how my eye was dilating.

What are good memories. Those reflections of moments when you knew someone cared. Someone would be there when you just need a hug or a shoulder to cry on. What's the use of retracing a lover, knowing that he'll never be back to take you in his arms, filling your soul with ecstasy? I have these vivid moments to gain a new knowledge of a current situation, as well as reminding myself that, I did it once, who's to say it might not happen again. The personal reminders that someone loved me once only gives me hope that someday romantic love may come again.

He worked as a housekeeper during the years 1985-1987. Micheal W. is his name and he resembled Kenny Rogers, yet slightly heavier. There was talk that he was 'gay' because he lived with a guy who also worked there and claimed to be 'gay'. Micheal and I would talk while he cleaned my sink or scrubbed my tub. He would take breaks when he knew I could go outside with him.

I came home from church one a Sunday. It was a beautiful day out, and I kept rolling in and out in order to catch glimpse of Micheal cleaning a bathroom or sweeping the dinning room floor. I didn't notice the letter lying on my bedroom table until after dinner. I read it twice to be sure the words he wrote were real. Micheal wrote of the love he had for me. The letter also said that he would be leaving me soon, but would be back and then we would never part. I thought he was insane! On that Sunday afternoon, I rolled into the dinning room just as he finished the floor. I noticed he was gazing in my direction, as if he had something he wanted to say but couldn't. We found we were staring at each other, and then he briskly walked over to me and kissed me on the lips. I still recall that moment so vividly, as if it had only happened yesterday!

I must have written Micheal twice a week, since staff or other residents were forever interrupting us. He didn't write back as frequently, but while we sat together during his breaks, Micheal kept talking as if we would never part. I remember waiting for hours, in our parking lot, for him to come and take me away from this maddening home. In all, he stood me up three times. Micheal seldom had a phone, which meant I could never call him to see where he was.

He did take me to his house once for pizza and pop. It was strange! Micheal and I were alone and both of us felt extremely nervous, almost as if we finally reached Heaven and were startled at the wondrous beauty of it all! He was a complete gentleman. When he smoked, he would stand in the doorway of his porch. We sat and talked until after 11:00 PM. when I said I must get home. He only lived five minutes away, which made the drive too brief. The moon was bright, and full of passion those only lovers understand.

The housekeeping staff gave me a surprise birthday party at Michael's house one year. This has got to be a fantasy of every sane woman who ever dreamt of a warm, romantic evening. There I was, sitting by a blazing fire with candles lit on the mantle. Micheal sat beside me all through that evening and, if there hadn't been six other people, we might have kissed again. We might have tenderly embraced to feel the sensation that two lovers find in a passionate moment! This was several years ago and yet I still dream of the day he will come back for me. I can still envision him in my doorway or working around Echoing Hills. In all reality, we may never meet again yet it's those memories that keep telling me that someone once loved me! Who's to say that moment was merely a taste of what was to come? He is merely a wonderful memory that will never be again. The last time I saw him was November 3, 1986. Some people really never fade from my heart.

Chapter 8

The Transformation

If I ascend up into heaven, thou art there:
if I make my bed in hell, behold, thou art there.
If I take the wings of the morning, and dwell in the
uttermost parts of the sea;
even there shall thy hand lead me, and thy right hand shall hold me.

Psalms 139:8-10

Given opportunities, a soul can soar into this orb with a sense of self-worth! Recognition of priceless riches that live deep within the frame of each being strives to get out. I was given that opportunity, one Saturday, when I moved out of Planceville Center with Deb. A research project began May 14, with two high functioning women, and many professionals said it would never work, We were only physical disabled! We were not mentally retarded! The lives, we each have, are limited to 70 or 80 years! I spent some sixteen years, and eight months, trying to get out of time schedules, restrictions in where, when and how long I accomplish any endeavor I may wish to participate in! I'm now finding some guidelines are essential in living as any able-bodied individual does. Here's how the next phase of my life came about.

Dear Mom,

How are you? Well, the summer of '93' is almost a memory! This has been an extremely busy season for me. I finally have my annuity started. That only took eight months and a lot of headaches. I found that the government made a mistake and still owe me twenty-five hundred dollars, which I can't get until I file income tax next year. I shopped till I dropped. They only gave me thirty days spend a little over eighty-one hundred dollars, so I got much of my new house furnished, besides a new wheelchair. I have my things in a storage lot now but tomorrow I'm going to talk with someone about storing my things on grounds after September 2nd. My actual moving month is January '94'.

I went up to Toledo on the 20th of July. We looked at three houses that afternoon. Ann, the girl who was going to share this house with me, also came with her case manager, and another case manager. I did think this was a bit strange, for Monica was Ann's case manager [and at that time mine] but I couldn't think why Karen, the second case manager was there until we were all sitting in the livingroom of the second house we looked at. Monica brought up having a third housemate. Ann loved this concept because this would cut down on living expenses and she is more concerned with going shopping and whatnot. We decided to go meet Deb the next day.

Ann had me over for supper that evening, yet hardly spoke to me. I explained why I didn't want a third housemate, and that made her uptight. Thank God Maggie, my driver/staff, was with me or that supper would have been a total flop! We talked back and forth since Ann was more interested in talking to her staff.

Maggie and I picked Ann up the following morning, and got lost trying to find the nursing home that Deb was living in then. I tried to make small talk with Ann, again, but she wouldn't talk. We were about an hour late and Ann's ride was at the nursing home already. Monica said she would bring Ann back some time the following week. Monica and I started talking about my previous night's experiences, and she agreed that Ann and I didn't belong together.

When I finally met Deb, it was like talking with a long lost friend! She was forty years old, with a BA in psychology. She was a quadriplegic and lived on her own out in California. We kept talking and making plans about the second house I looked at. She had to go into a home when she came back to Ohio because there were no Independent Living situations at that time. We agreed to be roommates without Ann. In my meeting, that very afternoon, I got through all my care plan paperwork, and then some big shot said that the board was slightly surprised that I wanted Deb, instead of Ann! In the beginning, way back in January, Shelly, who works at the Ability Center, told me I would have only one housemate. I didn't want two roommates! By golly, they listened. Deb saw the house and she loved it! I am learning not to let people walk all over me. We will move into our house this coming January. I can't wait!

Well, take care. Thank you for the plate. How was your trip? I pray to hear from you soon.

Shelly P. is the main reason I had the opportunity to move back to Toledo. I am very grateful to her for allowing me to come into this project.

November 22, 1993

Dear Shelly,

Merry Christmas! Christmas is each day of the year, if you think about it. I just wanted to say thank you for believing in me! You are a large reason that I have a house in Toledo. I will be living at the Planceville Center starting the first week of December.

On my four-day trip Deb and I looked through sales catalogs, and we interviewed four agencies for future staff. The interviewing process for staff took four hours. We picked an agency called 'Sunset Children's Home'. Don't be fooled by their name, for they used to only have a home for Physically Disabled. Now, they help the Supported Living Program by looking for people who want to be staff, and then Deb and I will interview those people.

I had to move up to the Planceville Center, where Deb had been living three years, until our house would be ready for us to move into. On December 18, 1993, Maggie drove me up to Toledo, with all my earthly possessions. That trip took three and a half-hours.

Why is it so frightening? I'm not myself now, and feel as if I didn't belong there? You are the main reason that I am finally going to live, as I want, not what someone else wants me to be! Take care!

December 19, 1993

Dear Maurice, (Maurice is the name I gave my computer.)

It's hard to believe I'm here now! I had breakfast in bed all three mornings, and I still go to bed by 9:30 each night. The thought of my house is helping my depression. My family's coming next Sunday for Christmas. Six more days till, people say, our Lord was born. What am I missing? This has been a dream of mine for seven years. Maybe I am just missing being known around town or I fear what is ahead of me? The people here are very good to me so why do I feel like crying?

December 20, 1993

Dear Maurice,

This has been a day to beat all days! I was on the go from 10:45, when I finally got up. I went to the activity room, to see about reserving a room for the Schauder Christmas and then some lady started an evaluation on me. She didn't get far because Kim, a staff member, came to get me for the house doctor.

Now, he's not your normal nursing facility doctor. He was eating meatballs when I came into his office, which was getting ready for a Christmas party. I thought, "You better not put me on a diet after I watched you eat in front of me." I just found out he increased one of my pain pills. Then the Occupational Therapy interrupted my Bible study to say that I'm too high functioning for their program, so she's calling Karen Howard (another case manager) to see if Specialized Services can help me.

December 23, 1993

Dear Maurice,

I cried today because I feared everyone I know suddenly went on vacation. Shelly never did come by and, when I finally called her, she was on Christmas holiday! I guess, if I ever move again, it won't be during the holidays.

I am embarrassed! I have Tony tonight! He's a very good staff at Planceville Center, yet I'm not used to a man handling me. This will be a change!

December 25, 1993

Dear Maurice,

And so this is Christmas! My last one in a nursing facility! Deb has been in bed, sick, since last Friday and I'm getting concerned. Christmas should be every day of the year, for Christmas is a feeling we get each time we go out of the way to do something for someone else. It's that joy you get when you make a new friend!

Today, Sue, my roommate at that time, told me the difference between a house and a home. A house is just a place where you keep your hat and coat! A home is where you feel the warmth of that hat and coat without wearing them! Sue had long black hair and was extremely wise. She had been a schoolteacher before a major stroke placed her here.

December 28, 1993

Dear Maurice,

I saw my first bout with death, after all this is an old folk's home. I shouldn't label the people who resided at Planceville Center; yet, many would live 70 to 96 years! There are some young people, but around there, they were the minority. Mary S. passed away, and I saw her family take her things away.

Mary lived in the room across from Deb. Deb was still in bed. I was getting concerned.

January 1, 1994

Dear Maurice,

Happy New Year! I wrote Maggie today. It was my second contact with Echoing Hills since I came on December 16th. I met a guy last night who reminds me of Chip. [Now, there was a sex fanatic]. Chip was a resident, at Echoing Hills, who thought he was God's gift to women. We met by way of phone and he lives across the street in Ashland Manor. His name's Bruce and he's only two years younger then me!

Jerry was my teacher at Ann J. grade school. We kept in contact over the years through birthday and Christmas cards. Here's a letter that I wrote him shortly after moving to Toledo.

January 5, 1994

Dear Jerry,

Happy New Year! How are you? You were my favorite speech therapist, and a fantastic trumpeter. It's hard to believe that I'm starting a new life! I moved up to the Planceville Center on December 16th and I'm already known as 'Trouble'. I can't wait till April! I just turned forty years young and I'm already living in an antique age home.

I never forget your birthday is the 6th of February. I tried calling you for your anniversary, but you were possibly in Spain doing some kind of a Mexican hat dance or sailing down some romantic river with Claudia feeding you grapes! It'll be over forty years that I've known you! Man, what a life we lead!

The Planceville Center isn't too bad of an institution. The food may leave something to be desired, yet the people care! Deb lives in another hall but she deals with being here by staying in bed all the time.

January 7, 1994

Dear Maurice,

Well, I made it three weeks and one day! They started remodeling our house. Deb is an extreme loner. She has been in bed ever since I came! It's odd, living with people who are either waiting to meet our Lord or wanting to die! April can't come soon enough!

January 11, 1994

Dear Maurice,

Julia died this morning at 7:40. I rolled past her room many times to say hi. She was a beautiful lady. She had some kind of muscle disease. Tonight, I called my Aunt Margie to tell her that I am in Toledo now. She reminded me that grandma lived just down the road. I reminded her that Uncle Jim did too.

After talking with Margie, I rolled around the first floor dining room, and their big screen TV had the 6:00 news on. They were interviewing a gentleman, who lives on Upton Ave. Grandma lived on that street for almost all her life, until they had to put her in a nursing facility

January 13, 1994

Dear Maggie,

The weather is cold and gray! Today is my one-month anniversary. It seems like longer, but it's not. It takes over a half-hour to answer a light! My roommate, Juanita, has it bad, because she has the backdoor trots!

Juanita and I are having bathroom problems with the two old ladies next door. They are in there eight times an hour! Granted, I only use the bathroom one-time daily, but they objected to my washing up in our bathroom, remember that is my only time in the blank bathroom. That institution's social worker wanted to put me on a schedule but I put my foot down on that concept! I have breakfast in bed every morning, then my coffee kicks in. I put my light on by 9:15, if I'm extremely lucky, I get on the throne! (Toilet) Well, for the past two days, somebody came to see me while I'm still trying to do my thing! Boy, a woman could get constipated at this rate.

Yesterday, I got all excited because my staff said a man was at my door! Here it was only a Jehovah witness. Man, this guy is really pushing his luck! This was the second time we met, and yesterday he started talking like I am sick! Well, I began to preach to him. He still said, "May I see you next week?"

Now, it's after supper and I'm hungry! I ordered the alternative, which was on the board as tuna noodle casserole, but came to my table as the cabbage and noodles that we had two nights ago! Boy, that cabbage leaves a lot to be desired. Tony, the staff feeding me, asked if I wanted my banana. I replied, "It's probably hard!" By golly, it was!

Planceville Center has a nationwide foot doctor who does room service. He came, while I was on the pot this morning, which was my second interruption. He's nice yet, I'm just another ten toes to him. Are you getting ready for the Valentine's dinner yet? I guess we have one too. One thousand eight hundred and forty-eight hours till I move into my house! They are carpeting it now, and putting a very high tech alarm system in it.

January 26, 1994

Dear Maurice,

Well, it could be worse. Juanita is moving to another place next week. I will miss her. Deb is doing something odd by not even wanting me to pass her doorway! I realize she's a very private person yet, they tell me that by my passing her doorway, and I'm invading her privacy. I tell you, I do not understand that woman. I think people stick their noses into things that aren't any of their business. If Ray, the institution's social worker, would let Deb and I learn how to live with each other without his guidance, we might be fine.

I met a new friend last Sunday. Janet is her name and tonight she brought her husband [Randy] over to meet me. They want to take me to Grace church Sunday. Janet found out that my house is three or four blocks from Larry E.'s house.

Leo B. was a professional lecturer on love and life, during the time I lived at Echoing Hills, and I collected all his books. I corresponded with him a few times, while I was in Planceville Center.

February 2, 1994

Dear Leo,

Happy Valentine's Day! How are you? Well, this nursing facility is certainly different than my old Echoing Hills! I meet more death, and see how many antique people can be very mean. One evening, at supper, a lady looked across the table at me and said, "I'm glad I wasn't born like you!" I kept thinking about how I want to grow old. It's not as easy as it seems. Think of all your friends that will escape this life before you and how many tears you will shed?

This Valentine is taking much more time than planned. Deb is a very unique lady. She has been hiding in her bed ever since I moved here on December 16th. Deb is highly private, and people tell me that I'm threatening her because I'm a very motivated person. I have been rolling on ice for a few weeks now. I'm advised to ignore her and wait till she speaks to me. Leo, that's not my personality! I'm doing it out of fear of losing our house. Ray, the social worker of this facility, wants us to be roommates when my current roommate moves out.

Well, take care?

As you may recall, Chris was an orderly at Echoing Hills, and ended up as a professional singer on an ocean liner down south. I wrote him after moving to Toledo.

February 8, 1994

Dear Christopher,

How are you? Happy Valentine's Day! Love is revealed to each being, on earth, in various ways. Much of love depends on how the receiver accepts this critical sensation. I fell in love with a church that believes in me! Now, don't get me wrong. I'm not religious! I only believe in God. You told me of your belief in an inner peace last August. Well, that's all very good, if you want that. I demand much more!

I require sunshine on a rainy day. Roses in the depths of winter. My case manager told me yesterday that I expect too much out of people. Well, why would you want anything less? I am getting my house, in spite of what Deb does! Deb might back out on this adventure. When I first met Deb, she was very open and eager to move. Since I moved here I learned that Deb is extremely private! She stays in herself and hides in bed all the time. I am moving, maybe sooner than April 1st. Now, who my housemate will be, is up in the air, but I still have a house!

Well, my friend, keep singing your songs. Take care.

February 10, 1994

Dear Maggie,

How are you? I miss you so very much, but I only have 1176 more hours until Wicklow is ready for two wild and wonderful women! Deb finally opened up to me Wednesday and boy, did she ever misunderstand me way back in August! This is the reason she's been avoiding me. I so much want to tell you what she thought, but she doesn't want anybody to know of her great misunderstanding! It scares me but, at least, I know what was troubling her.

Happy Valentine's Day! Love can be mistaken for something very immoral, against the word of God. My roommate moved out Monday. They wanted Deb to move in with me but she didn't want to damage our relationship. That was before we talked. Now, I have a little woman by the name of Jean, she's in the hospital right now for depression. They think I will keep her spirits up.

Well, have to go for now. Tell everyone hi!

March 8, 1994

My dearest Christopher,

Thank you for paradise. Actually, paradise can be a state of mind! Each time I think of you, I reflect upon the moments when we shared dreams and obstacles, which got in our paths of life. I recall when you fell in love and, deep inside my soul, I was furious. I guess this is a confession. Did you ever find a "someone" to care about? I'm still waiting, and praying, for mine. Up here, at Planceville Center, it seems like people only care because they get paid to do so.

I have twenty-four more days until I will be in my house with my own backyard and front door! I'm not sure of the outcome of this adventure, yet, I won't turn back now! It's memories, such as you, that keep me going. I remember that last dinner we had and how we opened up completely to each other. I miss that sort of paradise! Then, as we walked/rolled back to the car, there was a beautiful moon looking down at us. Oh yes, we both took unknown paths, but you're very close to me right now!

Well, my love, it's almost another spring! Another season to gaze up and see others walking, side-by-side, and arm-in-arm. Ah, but each spring is a new beginning for roses to bloom, suns to raise, and life to be lived! Write when your soul needs a friend.

March 12, 1994

Dear Leo,

How are you? This is a bigger transitional period for me than I thought it would be. I feel that I have to explain away my whole life-style because I happen to have a physical challenged existence. The church, that I want to belong to, asked me to write on Cerebral Palsy. Well, I did, then I got to thinking, why? Can't people accept me for who I am, instead of whom they want me to be?

My house will be finished tomorrow, yet we won't move in until some time in April. We are applying for a government-funded program that might not be ready until May 1st. You see, our moving date has been moved six or seven times now. I pray they won't delay it again.

Well, take care. I love writing you because you seem to understand. Spring is on its way!

Dear Maurice,

Larry and Halla were both residents of Planceville Center. Larry was only living there because he had lost both of his legs and could not find anywhere else to live. Halla was around eighty and was simply loosing her mind. Last night I helped Larry rescue Halla. Halla is around seventy and is very confused. She rides up and down these halls talking to people who live in her mind. She came down my hall and took off all her clothes and proceeded to turn the corner and roll away. Meanwhile, Larry was rolling up my hall. "Hey babe!" He always greets friends that way. I stopped him and warned him there was a nude woman around the corner. He didn't believe me until I showed him. He blocked her way while I ran to get the robe that she put on the knob of an office door. Larry put the robe back on Halla while I took her nightgown back to her station.

April 2, 1994

Dear Maurice,

It's the night before Easter, and I'm alone and still at the Planceville Center. This is my last holiday in a nursing facility. I saw "Beaches" for the third time on the TV in the resident's lounge this afternoon. Between the antique people screaming, and the staff talking among themselves, I had a good cry.

My roommate now is a sweet lady who can't talk. Betty T. is her name and she is a widow of five years. She had a stroke and wasn't able to live on her own anymore.

April 9, 1994

Dear Maurice,

Nattie won't be back. She's now living on a breathing machine. She lived about four doors down the hall and sat in a lounge chair all day, and all night. I will miss her. I heard she really didn't want to go to the hospital last week. Could she have known, in her mind, that she wouldn't be back?

Deb went into the hospital Thursday because of her bowels. Our moving day has been moved, once again, to May 9th. I'm beginning to disbelieve any date.

April 17, 1994

Dear Maurice,

A very beautiful mother died tonight. Mrs. Lee met the Lord shortly before 8:00 PM. leaving four children and a husband. Mrs. Lee had cancer at the young age of forty-three. A four-year-old lost her Mom and really can't understand death yet.

Deb came home Friday. We're going to interview staff starting tomorrow. Our moving date is now May 14th. I really can't wait!

And now, I must speak openly of the staff and residents of Planceville Care Center. I knew this would only be a short stay and so, I hoped not to get attached to too many people, but it's hard when you spend a quarter of a year here. I saw many residents come, and too few leave, alive to resume their own life story. What did I expect from an old aged home? This went on for sixteen years, eight month and thirteen days. That part of life is but, a few pages of a history book now! I really wonder why God kept me in an institution for so long.

And suddenly, my dream became reality! My own life started on that sunny Saturday morning. Instead of watching others build their bridges, I began to do what God called me to accomplish. Aspire to bring to this orb the talents that God has bestowed on me. If society binds each soul to what is in the written word, then, how does reality come about?

Supported living is quite different than existing in a nursing facility! I had a lot more responsibility. Deb and I felt controlled. I mean, not every household follows menus! If we were to manage all segments of our life, shouldn't we have more say in the staff who does our generic care? You may reply, "Oh, but we are paying them!" That's all well and good but you didn't see them on a daily basis, as we did! You never knew how well they work together, or how it felt, when someone came in with an attitude.

May 20, 1994

Dear Maurice,

Well, day six of my new life is extremely eventful. Before I even got out of bed, our alarm system went off three times. Last night, the telephone man arrived at 7 PM. He was due at 8 A.M. He checked out my phone jack and found that nothing was wrong with it. I felt like a real jerk! I called Carol W. about 8:30 PM., and it worked great. (Carol W. was my main nurse when I had my two spine operations in 1979.)

Did you know that the phone man gets eighteen dollars for every fifteen minutes? We were in the middle of supper so we asked him to come back in the morning. The following day, I turned on my clock radio, to dress to the morning show with Mark and Windy, when our alarm system went off. Pretty soon, firemen were at our door and 911 was ringing. Nancy, our staff, had to call Sunset and tell Barbara what happened. Did I tell you that my call button was accidentally pulled out of the wall Tuesday night? Since it was out of the wall, we taped the small alarm switch to the rail of my bed. Anyway, the alarm went off five more times before 8:00 A.M. I was going crazy! Gail S. came tonight and brought supper. I'm homesick! (Gail was my occupational therapist at Echoing Hills.)

May 21, 1994

Dear Maurice,

Day eight of my new life found me crying over my breakfast. Nancy showed me the blueprint of the next two weeks. Barb, the manager, has this week OK, but our third week gives us only fourteen hours of care a day. Now, our program [Waver 7] states we will get sixteen hours a day. I pray Barb will fill in those missing hours.

June 4, 1994

Dear Maurice,

It's 9:30 PM. on our third Saturday night. I went shopping, for food, in Sunset's van. Nancy, one of our staff at that time drove and my wheelchair went where the passager seat was. Barb, who was our supervisor of our house, decided it will go back Monday. We met our other neighbor tonight, a very good talker.

July 3, 1994

Dear Leo,

Happy 4th of July! How are you? I have been in my house since May 14th. It's a beautiful home, in a well-off neighborhood and I'm doing a lot of housework.

I really need your advice from this letter. I have a problem. I'm learning that, in order to be truly happy; I have to depend on my own self! The years spent in nursing facility only told me that I was leaning on others for my own contentment. [Very bad move] Now that I'm in a new living arrangement, I'm finding loneliness is encircling my very being! It's almost like living alone, because Deb doesn't get out of bed much. It's her life!

I eat alone. I do housework alone. Mange our house and purchase the household items needed to maintain it. I was told we were to share expenses, yet Deb takes her time when paying me back. Christ would give and give and then start giving! Deb wants separate cupboards. Doesn't sharing a house mean sharing responsibilities?

I guess it's the solitary way of Deb's life-style that makes it extremely hard to not share in the loneliness. I want to go places and do things! I want to live life and she is extremely private. I wanted this new life for so long and now it's like living on my own. Love was granted to us to share with the world. Each soul is lost, in one way or another and until we gain real friendships, we are but stray dogs trying to sniff out our next meal.

The great news is I'm cooking more since I'm out of a nursing facility. I made chili, baked a cake, and made various kinds of salads and a steak dinner. I'm waiting for your cookbook to come out so I can buy a copy. I'm also washing dishes, sweeping floors, answering the phone and door, as well as taking the sheets off my bed. If you knew how much I love it, Leo, I wonder how I existed in a nursing facility?

Well, my great friend, I must go for now. Take care of your soul. Remember we love the beauty of life!

Dee, another roommate I had at Echoing Hills, was born with Arthrogryposis. This disability restricts her arms and legs from bending. She is African-American and does everything with her mouth. Dee does her homework in bed on her stomach as well as needlepoint and paint. We had many fun times together. She moved out of Echoing Hills, and into her own apartment. Here's a letter I wrote her shortly after I moved into my first house.

July 10, 1994

Dear Dee,

Happy Birthday! I know it's early, but I have a lot of realizations to write you. I miss the chance to do something for your birthday (on August 6th), so I may bore you to death with the Wild, Wonderful undertakings of the Wicklow Woman! How's Rinda doing? How's the workload at Hopewell? Is Dave and Jean married yet?

I applied for the Governor's Counsel again, and now I'm about to get a seat on the board of P Squared. Let me explain: P Squared is the title of the housing project I live in. It stands for Preferred Properties. You would go crazy over my landlord (he's very handsome). Anyway, I'm on a barrier free committee, which meets once a month. I'm about to call our Mayor concerning my neighborhood, because I live right behind a mall but getting into the mall itself is extremely difficult! Once I'm in the mall, it's barrier free, but I take a chance on my life every time I try to enter it.

So, how's your love life? I have met some nice drivers on the Walker vans. Walker is only for medical appointments. They went out of business, so I found another transportation system, by the name of Brookside. We have another van system known as Tarps, but they want two-week notices.

Take care.

Sometimes, images from the mind never turn out exactly how you dreamt them to be. We were only allowed one staff person per eight-hour shift. Nancy, Hannah or Carlene worked the morning shift. A typical day begins at 6:30 A.M., when Hannah would wake me up. Actually, it was my choice what time I got up. While I did my thing, used the bathroom, she went to give Deb her suppository and then she came back to take care of me. If I was ready to get up, Hannah will sponge bathe me and get me up. She would fix my breakfast, which I directed what I wanted to eat. As she fed me, Hannah wrote a list of what I needed to accomplish for that day. Then, she gave me my morning medications.

When Deb woke up, Hannah would do her medication and see what she wanted for breakfast that morning. After she got Deb situated for a while, Hannah brushed my teeth and combed my hair. We had a new rule about transferring me on the toilet for a BM because too many of our staff had hurt their back pivoting; they used a manual lift on me. That lift is a new concept for me, and not quite a joyful experience in itself! Hannah looked in on Deb while I was on the toilet to see if she wanted anything. After taking me off toilet, Hannah started cleaning up the kitchen and fix Deb's breakfast. While feeding Deb, she would give medication to her. Then, Hannah would bath Deb and got her up if she wanted, try to encourage her anyway. It was almost like living alone, because Deb didn't want get out of bed much. It was her life!

Hannah brushed Deb's teeth and combed her long black hair. Then, whoever was working that day finished cleaning the kitchen and made our beds. If there were wash to do, they would help me get it done. By that time, it was my lunchtime, so Hannah fed me while working on a list of things to be done for that day. We would forever have things for one our staff to do on and off through out the day. The key concept is working whatever into the schedule. Before they go home at 1:30 PM., they would put me on and off the toilet, and give 2:00 PM. medication. If I had a good book, Hannah would put it on the side of the dining table closest to kitchen, along with my large cup of ice water with the TV remote at its side. Making sure we had everything we needed for the next two hours, Hannah left for the day.

The evening was uniquely lonely for me. When Nancy came, she would help me with the bathroom, after she gave Deb a drink. When Deb stayed in bed, she ate first and then I try to think of something quick and simple to make, because Deb called her back to her bedroom every ten minutes. I bought TV diners in order to eat quickly. Deb ate extremely light. If she would eat, it might be three chips with avocado dip. I worked on Maurice or watched VH1. I went to bed around 10:00. I used the lift when I got into bed, and finished watching TV.

A counselor had me write down everything that frustrated me for about three years. He worked ten minutes from my house. Deb never appreciated me expressing my independence. I started going to him because of my frustration with Deb. She hardly came out of her room, and when she did, it was either for doctor's appointments or Sundays, when her dad would carry her from her bed to his car. It was as if her entire family never accepted her disability. She broke her neck the night before her prom and never really got over not walking. I thank God I never walked. She was trying to starve herself and her meals were few. Her dream finally came true on March 26, 2000 when she past away from Pneumonia.

I had just moved around the block onto East Lincolnshire Jan. 9, 1999. I needed to move away from Deb, because we just didn't see eye-to-eye anymore. I applied for a new home and two roommates. Finally, the management of the housing project that I live under found a house just around the corner. At first, they told me that I could move in July of 1998. Then, they said September and then December. It was a very foolish thing to do, but they kept prolonging the moving date. My new house was all ready, so I rode over in my chair and wouldn't go back.

This all began about four years ago at Barry's Bagels. I needed two roommates, at that time. Paula was low functioning but needed to get into Supported Living. She used to live at Maryland Nursing Home and refereed to that as "The Jail". When we met she was fifty-five and used an electric wheelchair. She used to follow me around this area. Her sight got bad. I recall one time I lost her. I came back to the house crying. She was always super slow and I nicknamed her Pokey. Paula laughed all the time and enjoyed church activities and shopping. Paula and I went to Westgate and saw the Grass Roots, among other musical groups. We didn't get home till 11:45 PM. The Young Animals were going to be down there the following evening. Paula knew that we needed a third roommate, so she asked me if I would meet her girl friend, Karen. She also lived at Maryland Nursing Home, but she's ambulatory, and loves to do crosswords and enjoys eating Chinese. Karen doesn't require any physical care. She had to move to another house, which doesn't need 24 hour staff, on December 26, 2002.

As our life enters this world, so must we depart. Paula was a non-insulin-dependent diabetic, and cancer ran in her family. She had to go back to the ER, because her sugar got too low again. I got so mad at her because she would always call me Bozo, but now I am very mad at myself for getting mad at her. She past away on Sunday, January 12th at 2:00 in the afternoon, and I still can picture her laying there in a three-piece pants suit in a casket.

The whole west side of Toledo knew me now. In rainy, snowy bad environmental factors I stay in my house, in my office. This is where I do my writing. Well, where do I begin to tell you what a full life I have now? I shall go by the days of the week. By the way, this is being typed on my new computer. I have E-mail now which keeps me busy. I'm a member of Washington Congressional Church five blocks from my house. I went each week except days friends came down or up, depending on where they're coming from. In the afternoon I would go down to my hot spot, Barry's Bagels. I know almost all the staff even Barry himself! Mondays I normally go to my bank and to the Foodtown, near to my house. Barry's built a higher table, because my seat is higher than their tables, so that's where I eat out and get all the coffee I want for one low price!

A time back, each Monday and Friday I swam at the Anne Grady Center, which we hire our staff from. I had two instructors, Heather and Shelly. Connie, who was my day staff then, usually went on Mondays, and she walked with me very well in the pool because she is tall. She also swam under water and likes goofing around in the pool. I have a lot of arthritics in my body and it's very difficult to get stage four sleep, which is the most important for your organs. God never gives us more than we can bear! I'm in constant pain because I developed Lupus in November of 1998, which is pain in the muscles all the time.

Tuesday evenings, I pulled our trashcans to the curb, anticipating Wednesday's garbage pick-up. The following morning, I would pull them back up to the side of our house, before going to get my weekly allergy shot. I have been going since May of 1997, and now the staff feels like family to me. I'm very comfortable with my doctor. I nicknamed him Hairy, because he is bald and he's forever talking about how bad I drove my wheelchair to their office, Ann and Lynn were his nurses, and they gave me my shots. I have a very poor immune system and need IVs every three weeks. This can take up to four hours. Ann's very good at getting a vein on the first or second try. I have deep veins, from my dad. Betty the receptionist was a hard egg to fry. Each time I accidentally hit the wall with my chair, she would quiver as I made another nick in the woodwork. She is going to buy a skateboard and hold on to my handlebars while we roll around the West Side of Toledo. She's my beautiful old lady! I would feel lost if I never found these people. We are a close knit family of strangers. Thursdays I worked on my computer with Sariah.

My staff have almost all changed. Some for the better and a few who you wouldn't care to see again. I'm cooking more often! I cracked eggs for a cake, once, and I saw my first flying yoke! I have made chocolate chip cookies and pizza! I make a mean microwave dinner. I open the box and put it in the microwave all by myself! I enjoyed cooking with one of my staff Rena. Rena Mae was here when Paula was living. Rena's the best cook we have now. She puts Betty Crocker to shame. She nicknamed me 'Sugar-Lips'. Don't ask me why. Rena's half of the 'Dynamic Duel'. I call her and Sheri that because they work well together on the afternoon shift. They talk like an old married couple. Sheri really has an ability to make me feel well about myself. We had Diana who never slept. She was going to school to become a nurse and is a single mom. It took me a long time but I can really say that I admire her for her determination to follow her dream, no matter how much Hell this society gives her.

Lashauna usually worked 11:00PM. Till 7:00A.M. She wasn't feeling good and had to be on light duty for a while. She's a unique woman! You'll find a lot of back problems in when working as a personal care staff. Christy was our team leader, at that time, and I caught her bouquet at her reception, which means that I have to marry before February 9, 2003.

Karen had just moved out of our house December 27, 2003 so that left me in this three-bedroom range house on my own. I interviewed two other women. Kim was really cool. Only trouble was, she had to sell her house before she could move in with me. Christy introduced me to a low-functioning woman by the name of Julie who moved in on March 1, 2004. She has a lot of behavior problems that make me feel like I'm living with a time bomb.

Gloria who has a bedside manner like a Bobcat in heat. They moved her to another house. Rena's related to her by marriage, not by cooking, that's for sure. Cindy makes good coffee and likes the show that was called Big Brothers 3. Toni and Christine mostly work the night shift. Toni taught me to "Talk to the hand!" We would talk to the different body parts after a while. Christine tells me what she has been doing with her house. She's an accident waiting to happen. She loves cats. Sandy is my primary, which means she schedules all my doctor appointments, as well as keeping my medications stocked up. She's a good friend too. Amber's a lady of all talents and master of few, just like everyone on earth. She took my computer apart and put a DVD player in my computer. She is a student at Toledo University and teaches. She was one of my favorite staff, before she quit to get married at the end of October into an instant family.

Tracie will be our house supervisor starting September 1. She calls me Patrinca for some odd reason? She just got married and her new last name's Rock. I sing songs to her with the word Rock in them. Marty F. is the Director of Community Programs, the head of Supportive Living. He's bald and so I nicknamed him my Hairless-Wonder. Chris F. is Tracie's boss. He is over-seeing my house and makes sure my staff completes their paperwork. Gretchen, his wife, is proofreading my book for me. Similar to a nursing facility, Chris writes programs that we have to try to accomplish. One of mine is putting CDs into my computer. All the staff I ever had, had a gift of looking far beyond my four wheels and shaky limbs.

In many ways, I had a variety of families, isn't that like any person. That is why I wrote this book, to tell as many people as possible, that each person on this earth has something to offer.

Chapter 9

I wanted to include my poetry with the book to give further insight to my life and how I have expressed myself.

Poetry

Poems

"A True Friend"

As I ponder this life of mine I praise my Lord he brought to light
the sheer beauty of knowing you!
Two spirits ascended beyond reality to merely find
a time and space which was only in their mind.
Touch me with the beauty of your words
And come taste the flavor of my life's bittersweet wine!"
Life is a series of actual events that could set sail with any desire
turning a flicker of hope into a blazing fire!
That infernal ship which glides across every starry eyed lover
viewing that which practical minds ignore!
Never allow this norm to sweep these away laughing hysterically as if to say
"There's no need for you all flawed and weak!"
You pray for your finale as sorrow engulfs your very soul
yet in your weakest hour He is truly glorified!

If dreams are blocks on which you build your existence
Nourish those tiny sparks until new hope is born!
A friend is your soul's needs complete
to share the bitter as well as the sweet!
Why must we meet merely to become a part
knowing only too well that certain spark
may stay hidden deep within the walls of our hearts
if we never risked a "Hi!"
Within a split second an endless lifetime appears
when you challenge your all for the sake of a smile.
A soul sailing into the depths
to see the beauty of a thunderstorm.
A rose may never die if by chance one really does pray!
Accept the fact that many will run while few will actually care
about a dying rose or a grizzly bear.

Just a mere fraction of an endless time gone berserk
as two solitary souls soar deep beyond the sphere of a smile
to gain the entire ecstasy of a true friend!

"Church Bells"

Did you ever hear a deaf man sing as church bells rang out one day?

They sang a bittersweet tune to the town

that a father, sister, mother or brother departed from this road called life!

Accept the fact that in order to gain we must surely forfeit a friend or lover!

For in order for a rose to bloom it must first feel the rain.

Did you ever see a lame man fly or a diamond sailing towards the sky?

Reach out for a rose yet beware of its thorns

as time rushes on and someone else is born!

If by chance we venture once again deep within the core of another

don't fear what might not be there!

Accept the fact that many will run while only a few really care!

Touch me with the beauty of your words!

Hold me with a passionate smile until death knocks at my soul.

Until that moment when we shall become whole.

Did you ever hear those church bells weep

as little boys meet little girls and life goes on its why.

Oh Lord does it really pay?

How priceless is a friend like he

yet death has its means of shattering the physical.

The tangible evidence of a father, sister, mother, brother!

Did you ever see the beauty of a red rose die?

The church bells chimed yesterday for yet another spirit in the sky

as softness of night comes!

Must we fear the answers to why?

Accept the fact that love lives on even if those church bells ring.

"The Man in the Middle"

And there He hung.
No words left to be sung.
His life barley begun
when we mocked and cried,
"We must have Him die!
The man in the middle.
The one they call Christ!
Let's put Him to the test
to see if He will really
pay the price!"

He suffered for our sin.
He bled for our immorality
but never turned back.
Did the man in the middle
ever think twice?
He was pierced for our transgressions
and died a brutal death
yet He rose on the third day
so we will could never have to pay!
And there He hung yet many today
are still questioning
the reality of the man in the middle?

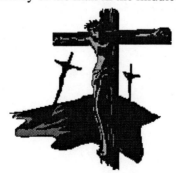

"Deep Within"

Upon a dream so long ago
I prayed to God someday we'd meet?
For deep within a tear stained night
I sang to Him the need to be!
The desire to expose all my life's fantasies
into the warmth of a lover so true.
Some may hear yet fail to understand
the frail awe that a greeting brings!
Combining the sorrow of yesterdays sadness
with hope for tomorrow's delight
and see how simple a vision takes flight!
Take me as I truly am,
for I may never change from black to white
or red to green and back again
No one will ever know how long this might last!
never actually considering the illusive past.
Reach out for a rose yet beware of its thorns.
Seek out that mystical love that binds two souls
into one beautiful friendship achieved by a "Hi"
Until that day when we will be totally whole!

"Toward the Sky"

Did you ever gaze towards the sky
forever pondering reasons why?
On a silent midnight when the moon was full
I closed my eyes and thought of you.
What is it when all your hopes
are crushed by society's mode?
Are all the ashes buried forever?
After the flames of a vision die
look towards the sky!
Never allow this norm to sweep goals away
laughing hysterically as if to say
"There's no need for you all flawed and weak!"
You pray for sleep as your sorrow engulfs your very soul!
Wait!
In our weakest hour He is truly glorified!
If dreams are blocks on which you build a life
why tarnish the beauty of my conceptions of my world?
Nourish those tiny sparks until new hope is born!
Ignites into a million little known facts called life!
If need be venture within the frame of my bitter being
to see anther's way.
To view the setting sun or a rising mourn
and thank the Lord for the day you were born.
What's life but several wrongs explaining away too many rights?
A battered sea gull trying to take flight
within the depths of a stormy night!
Did you ever ponder the facts of life
and accepting the way it has to be?
Gaze toward the sky and remember me?

"A Gift"

As I ponder this life of mine
I praise my Lord he brought to light
the sheer beauty of knowing you!
Two spirits ascended beyond ecstasy to merely find
a time and space which was only in their mind
A friend is your soul's needs complete
so I praise our Lord
He gifted me with you!
To share the bitter as well as the sweet!.
Why must we meet merely to become a part
knowing only too well that certain spark
may stay hidden deep within the walls of our hearts
if we never risked a "Hi!"
Why must the public eye dictate what each vessel sings?
When each babe has an unique quality
that desires nothing more than the best!
Her ship must sail both north and south.
East and due west!
In this certain space in time
caress my loneliness with gentle words of love!
Refresh my understanding with fields of joy
where life is simple and ever so sweet
A real friend is your soul's needs made complete!

Within each solitary self lies a beauty beyond compare
waiting to be nourished by someone like you!
Within a split second an endless lifetime appears
when you risk it all for the sake of a smile.
To know for certain a true friend is near!
A soul sailing deep within to see the beauty of a thunderstorm.

Venture into the realm of another not only reaching for a smile
but gaining the entire ecstasy of a true friend!
A rose may never die if by chance one really does pray!
Trapped in a world of stereotypes and bitter looks a friend is a friend
indeed.
I praise our Lord He gifted me with you!

"Smile"

At times I scale a mountain ever so high
pondering the magnet between you and I!
Why is it so agonizing to be my self
within this span of time
when you're unsure of the end of each rhyme?
Come closer and listen to my toneless song
to merely hear the sincere statement of a solitary soul
striving to sail beyond society's stares!
Gazing behind to notice no one there!
At times like these I search a silvery sea
to merely find life's reflections encircling me!
Be near me my friend,
for life's silhouettes are infinite to the taste
like Autumn leaves that sways through the crowded sky!
It matter not what shadow you cast
on a white wall sparkled black
as long as you're willing to venture a smile, a sigh,
a curious glance as you walk by!
If only for a mere wink from your eye
my soul could sail beyond each crowded sky
into the haven of your gentle arms
An endless reason to chance it all
simply to see if this one will last?
No one's absolutely right or definitely wrong
like the words to some instrumental love song!
Still society fails to understand
that a blind man sees much more than darkness can bear!
Come taste the fragrance of my dreams if you dare
for nothing's perfect if you neglect to chance!
In a soundless room does anyone care to dance!

I am who I am by the wondrous hand of God
so it's simply too bad if this norm labels me odd!
Come closer and listen to my toneless song
striving to feel as if this iron lace could actually belong?
And to each season comes a unlimited reason
to jeopardize everything for the sake of a smile!
Discover that magnet between you and me
instead of running in sheer disgrace
with that pathetic look upon your face!!
At a certain space in eternity's cycle
peace shall embrace this sincere soul.
So hello, my friend,
won't you enter and make me whole.

"Glory Land"

By the time I get to Glory land
a few more nights I will sit and cry.
A few more prayers I shall shout to the sky!
Why must we live merely to have each dream
shattered by society's means!
And the lightening flashed before my eyes
Why can't society see beyond my shell
instead of molding me into their mind's insight
Must I continue this nightmarish Hell
until my soul sets sail on a timeless trail.
When will they understand that no one really fails.

By the time I get to Glory land
a few more dawns I will wake still wondering why.
What am I searching for and how long might it last.
Why am I forever looking in the past.
Yesterday is dead and gone into the depths of eternity
as mere perceptions lay scattered in my mind
of soft smiles and tender sighs
before the bittersweet words of goodbye!
If I only listened with my heart
would we still be apart.

By the time I get to Glory land
a bit more knowledge I might understand!
I keep pondering if this is really His plan.
Why can't others see beyond my shell
instead of molding me into their mind's insight
of what a human must never be!'
By the time I get to Glory land

many more graves shall cover His space!
People will care less by the look on their face!
Is it money or fame.
A small child winning their first baseball game.
Life is too brief to keep running in disgrace!
Many more logical minds won't understand
the love You have for all the land.
A mighty oak can surely learn to bend!

"The Jar"

Silhouettes of smiles are kept in that jar by the door.
Shadows of what might have been
would have been if time wasn't so bitter.
Empty words echoing through out my mind
caring and sharing but yet walking away!
"Oh well, maybe yet another morn.
Might be on the day you were born."
A stain glass pain might blind the sun
yet a sightless eye views beneath the night!
Traces of joy are kept in that jar by the door.

Implications of entities that could have been
if dreams were nurtured and cared for,
like newborn babes in this world so cold!
Oh to be so bold!
Yet what is life,
but frequent hellos with endless good-byes.
Memories of what should have been if time didn't have its way.
Say what you mean and mean what you say!
Others will like you through out your day!
Isn't that way any friendship begins?

Indications of laughter in the face of shivering sorrows
are kept in that jar by the door.
Oh well better luck tomorrow.
If merely by a simple "Hi!"
my smile shall strive far beyond your serene wink,
and simple silvery sigh
we could become comrades in this life!
To reach for acceptance

but gain a lifetime camaraderie so true!
My soul needed someone like you

Risk into the realm of a smile
enabling that innermost being
to set sail on a chance!
Reach out for that magical love
which only two can touch with a soft "Hi!"
Whenever I'm down and feeling blue
I gaze toward that jar by the door
recollecting the times I thought I could fly
from talking with someone such as you!

"Bless Him!"

Bless Him for each ray that shines
on a cold winter's day like today.
Bless each small child
who glances at the sky
forever wondering why.
The silent friendship between you and I!
If only our souls could dance
to the glorious glory of natures song
Many shall find that they truly belong!
Come along and set sail on my song.

Bless Him for each soul I touch
and the knowledge of a spark divine.
Enhancing your soul thought out this life
as fine bittersweet wine!
Seek out your fortune merely to find
the search for true love will surely be found
if you'll reach towards Heaven
with your feet on solid ground.
Open your heart instead of your mind
to merely see many brick walls slowly bend.
Accept the fact that in order to truly gain
we must surely lose much more.
Recall that Friday morn someone died only to be born!
Reach out for a pedal yet beware of its thorns!

Bless Him for the open doors
as well as the ones that never do.
Bless Him for making my world anew!
For each star above on a moonlit night

as well as His loving grace
which saves me from fright!
For the neighbor next door who smiles with a hi!
Each golden souvenir of days gone by!
Reflections of long summer nights
with cod winter good-byes!
Of fresh spring souls that forever were there
whenever clouds sail across the sky.
Most of all bless Him for friends like you!

"Christmas is..."

A time to stop and think
of all the things we should be thankful for.
A time of joy and being happy.
Of giving to make others smile.
A feeling of warmth
when tender moments come for awhile.
To have that sense down deep inside
that a heart was touched,
because of you!
A time for people to look around and see all the priceless gifts
like the newborn baby down the road,
or that old-fashioned friendship
that could never be bought with gold.
A time of people who always care
for tears shed over a lost love affair!
A time of singing carols,
and screaming at the top of your lungs,
Merry Christmas to all and my love to you!
A time to build a snowman,
and counting flakes on your nose.
To bundle up safe and warm from your head to your toes!
A time to ponder what Christmas really means?
Not just new toys and an evergreen,
but the birth of our Lord on high,
and the saving grace for you and I!
Yes Christmas is many things to me,
as for how many drum sticks,
please pass me three?

"Beware"

Beware of yesterdays!
For thoughts of years back will bring sad memories
which shall only tell you what you might lack.
That only lead to tears falling from your eyes
as you realize that yesterday's dreams
aren't coming true today!
Oh well maybe tomorrow,
if it ever does come?

Beware of a hi!
For a million hellos
just mean a million good-byes,
and farewells are painful if they're from the heart.
Are you brave enough to open yourself to another
which may lead to love or a tragic adieu.

Beware of love!
For love stabs like a knife if it's real,
and not just a game two fools play!
Love is as beautiful as a sunset
yet so painful if you must let it go!
But if no feelings existed
then yesterdays would have no memories
and we couldn't have dreams that might come true tomorrow
if we have faith,
yet please beware?

"Rat Race"

Speak up
yet let no one hear.
For cares must wait
until all the endless paperwork is done.
Allow life's rat race to capture your mind
neglecting the need of a friend.
Resign to the fact that championships cost
time and money.
Still souls weep!
Recall Christ!
He gave His time as tears were shed
for the mere price of love.
Tenderness that has no tags
by which is told the worth of a soul.
Scream,
yet expect to wait for if need be
tomorrow your fears might be examined.
So carry on my friend and wait!
This rat race comes first,
before the time for a tear.
Before that love Christ gave
for time is money
yet still souls weep!

"Greenbacks"

Do you care that I weep?
That these painful tears
long for the warmth of a hug.
Hear the frightening screams
of a lonely child
craving for a gentle smile.
Would greenbacks mend
a broken heart or ease a lost soul.
Can money buy love
as a song on the radio sings.
What will I do
on a lonely night like this?
I'm broke!

"Hope"

Hope!
What is it, ·
when all your dreams are crushed by society's mode
are all the ashes buried forever?
After the flames of a vision die
look towards the sky!
Never allow this norm to sweep them away
laughing hysterically as if to say,
"There's no need for you, all flawed and weak!"
You pray for death as your sorrow engulfs your very self
but wait,
in your weakest hour
He is truly glorified!
If dreams are blocks on which you build a life
keep them!
Nourish those tiny sparks until new hope is born!
Ignites into a million little known facts
called life!
If need be
venture within the frame
of this bitter norm
yet never release that ray of hope!
For that ray was given by God
and God never fails
so why should you?

"Solitude"

Solitude
is the tender relationship
between your mind and soul.
It's the gentle sway of a leaf in springtime.
Of a child's smile when rewarded by a kiss.
Two lovers reuniting
to show that they were truly missed!
That inner eye which views
what logical minds ignore.
What is love but the unspoken word
screaming to be held
by someone like you!
It's stillness after a soft but sad goodbye.
That brief second in time
when reality halts lovers and they are no more!

Solitude is the knowledge
of yesterdays sinking into the depths of eternity
to never surface again.
The faith in God that tomorrow will bring
answered prayers and dreams.
It's the realization of memories stabbing your mind
until tears escape the innermost walls shouting, "It's over!"
Then it fades away granting you peace once again.
Solitude can be a lonely soul in search of warmth!
It hurts,
but at least I'm at peace with my mind!

"Mrs. K."

It's simple!
I'm created by God but stem from a cage.
Weep not,
for the aim of my being is not to be an object
as cats, rats and elephants.
Bound up by logical, practical ways, my soul cries out, Touch me!
Hold me through this endless night!
Feel this harsh reality making mincemeat out of my heart.
Frigid reasoning enslave my soul my hopes and desires
to 9 or 10 volumes of what mere man thinks life ought to be?

Look, no one knows the true meaning of why my limbs shake?
Why my words drip at times and the sun goes down at night?
No one but Him!
Minds sweep away each vision that fills my soul with joy!
For a dream is but a mere story told by the heart
yet not to be known around society's norm.
Must this go on?
My life is but a minute drop of rain upon His garden of forever!
My framework might defer from that of yours
but my soul longs for equality!

Hold me for each being on earth
strives for the warmth of another.
Touch me allowing your self to intertwine with mine.
Run with me,
for this fact was a dream just a moment ago!
Just as my soul cries out "I want to be free!'

"Timeless Meaning"

Walk,

leaving your sorrows behind

and climbing toward the high calling of God.

Let time race on to only gaze back to see you walking.

Don't allow the ticking of a clock to enchain your dreams

like some caged eagle praying to be free!

For what is time but a captor of your mind!

Sail with your dreams and see what you may find?

Forgive time for humans fabricated it.

They laugh at how moments rush by neglecting to love

or be loved during a lonely night.

They won't stop to notice the beauty of a gentle smile

or the tenderness of a silent tear.

Love!

Allowing the beauty of God

to shine within you to merely reflect

His loving kindness to solitary souls like me.

Give your spirit a chance to soar with memories gone pass

and visions that will surely last!

The heart brakes many a time

yet the soul remains solid as a tree against the wind.

Fly

leaving reasoning behind far from the practical brains

who can't see Him beyond the rain.

For the logical mind with its earthly ways are lost as to what is right?

Forever searching for the bow in the sky!

Journey over your pain to a life where hearts are free

without time to stop the wondrous feeling of love!
Yes my friend come fly with me
to see the true beauty of God
shining deep within you!

"Words"

Call them what they are
words are mere chained up syllables
which praise God's name as well as build hatred!
Why Lord?
Why can't these sounds
rejoice in Him instead of destroying decent souls
such as you and me.
Piercing like a knife until we pray to die!
No one really knows the answer
to the question of why?

Words!
They become the life of a party
or cut until one bleeds to death!
Yes clothe in knowledge the fearful terms of passion
may lead to nothing but a big lie!
They hurt and bend your mind so
that it's extremely tough to think.
Isn't that Satan's way?
Of bursting every dream you have until your world is null and void.
When all you hold is yesteryears.
Here comes the tears!

Stop!
Listen to a child at play neglecting these terms only big kids know.
Ah, to be a child again!
To laugh away these foolish sounds,
that kill your soul and ruin the love of God.
Oh, to be a child again!

"An Enigma"

The self!

That portion of your being,

which hungers to be heard,

craves to sing out, "Need me! Take me for who I am,

for that's all God intended me to be!"

Reveals itself to the public eye merely to be known by others,

yet must maintain an identity!

Like a seed longs for a soft spring rain,

to mature into God's excellence,

each heart must consider the connecting force!

Each enigma born to this earth,

must pay homage to the next link in line,

to fully understand the complexities of mortal man.

Come, take my hand!

The self!

That innermost being which makes someone unique,

dares to be a necessity!

A vital segment of this sea of life,

that screams to be heard within a deaf society.

A blind man sees by touch!

The mute observes each motion,

in order to grasp as much!

An enigma striving for significance cause,

yet longing to be loved,

on a cold abandoned obsession as this?

No being on earth is completely at bliss!

Be!

If arrogance doesn't blind your way,

causing pride to obstruct your day!

If the rose wilts from mockery and tainted tales

it's only your insane disdain,

keeping you for the rain!

If dreams are merely foolish prayers,

just echoing through a heart you will never sow that seed,

God planted within you and me!

It matters not what shape you inhabit,

for many will accept the rose,

that seed beneath the snow.

For they knew the gift God gave was you!

Sing to me your song of life and we shall see the glory of His love!

"Upon your Love"

Upon a moment so long ago
you viewed me with your very soul!
You stopped to see beyond my shell
only to remind me that I am really whole!
Why must we fear the things we most want?
Why must the rainbow fade away only to come back another day?
For as your eyes enfold the very sector
from which I gain courage to fight this endless struggle called life.
the promise of your soul softly shines.
Why do the stars show their glow only after dusk influences the day
to enter the depths of the night?
No greater love is there than that within your very self!
Come be my friend!

Upon a season so long ago I gazed beside to only find
a smile so gentle and ever so kind!
For through your eyes reality's ways
neglects to keep that certain drive back.
If you were a mountaintop
I would scale to your highest peak
to only touch the forever in you.
Ecstasy shall unfold the splendor of your jagged illusions of why you are you
and I'm merely me?
You felt the prism of light deep within this core of mine
to merely taste the bittersweet wine of a love that's divine!
Upon a kiss love took flight and that small spark
turned into a blazing flame!
Is it merely a chance few risk for the sake of the heart?
Give me your love and we shall truly never part!
"Forever"

In the still of a midnight prayer
visions of a priceless love
sailed gently within my mind and again I ask God why?
Why does each being crave to be held
as each setting sun ask only to become
the beauty of a full grown moon
dancing among the still soft stars.
And then He gave me you!
Be
for who you really are
is a reflection of God's love.
A gift sent from above
yet craves to be needed uniquely by me!

Ecstasy!
Each time we touch I gain a greater sense
of your desire to be only mine!
Come live only for this span of time for yesterdays are past
while tomorrows are simply dreams yet to be!
True love isn't bought or sold with money, silver or gold.
It is felt by soft hugs!
Passionate kisses that will never grow old!
And when our lips meet ecstasy will intertwine our souls
until we are together totally whole!
Oh what eternal bliss when forever will be ours
with merely a tender kiss!
Sing to me your soft songs of life for you are a prayer come true
which is why I'll forever love you!

"And to Each Season"

And to each season take a chance!
Allowing each vision
to fall into place like ice crystals.
If I was a snowflake
I would fall upon your nose
merely melting until I became a part of you!
Deep within a portion of my being
lives what the mere eye cannot view!
Does each insight have a need
to bend the mind and tear the heart?
To shred any tangible time that lovers may only kiss,
and then fearfully depart!
Let me look within myself
to only discover reflections of you.

If by chance our dreams might combine
to merely form a portrait of magnificent ecstasy
as the bittersweet taste of wild berry wine we would rejoice with vestal
friendship!
And to each season comes a unlimited reason
to jeopardize everything for love.
Never asking for a fall yet gaining what no mortal man can see!
Life is merely a series of actual events lingering within the core of you and me.
building until our final breathe!
Risk!
What becomes of love may never be fully known
until we will truly go home!
In this cold life of hateful stares.
People who talk yet really don't care
I praise God there's you!

"Your Fortune"

Seek out your fortune
and you may find that it just might take,
a matter of time?
An hour, a day,
a year, two decades?
Don't just establish a rut,
and watch as life's parade scurry on.
One needs a fire a blaze that burns!
Open up with a "Hi",
and a whole new venture you will learn!
Is it there in your eyes as we greet each day?
An inferno warming each soul with a smile!
Fools, pure idiot can't see beyond volume upon volume of forgotten lorn
that a brilliance blind to the naked eye
is igniting like a baby being born!
The beauty of a setting sun!
The enchantress of a full-grown moon fills my mind each time we speak,
as the frail wonders of a friendship brews into a priceless act of God!
A rose is a rose,
is a rose none can compare!
A tender, precious gem that only God could create
shall unveil itself to this orb if given the opening of society's door.
Harmony is all that's God implores to each heart on earth.
Nothing more!
Modern man fails to truly understand
the awesome wonder of God's gift to man!

"A Mere Moment"

It's such a small thing to greet the morning sun.
To feel the fresh Spring,
and live each moment as if it were the last!
Neglecting the fault of yesterdays and anything out of the past
It's such a microscopic entity to search for today's treasures!
A smile passing by or someone special singing "Hi!"
Any being can dream yet few have the innate urge,
to let reality hear its scream!
Allow me to listen to your dreams.

Why?
Why must the public eye dictate what each vessel sings?
When each babe has an unique quality
that desires nothing more than the best!
"Welcome to my world", sang a blind man one-day.
"Show me your sunset and I'll let you feel mine.
Come taste the flavor of life's bittersweet wine!"
"Come listen to my melody.", A mute monk exclaimed.
"God hears each whisper as well as each shout made
from high on top of any mountain."

It's such a slight second to view a full grew moon.
To touch the Autumn wind as leaves come tumbling down.
To love just for the joy of it!
Oh the times that were shall never be again,
so simply share the still soft seconds
before death marches through my door!

"Fire"

If only for a mere minute in time
could you taste my life's bittersweet wine?
Please don't reject me simply because the elite labels me odd!
Each being was born to thirst for another's warmth and weakness.
To search high and low for someone to share
a melancholy morning.
If merely to be near within the darkest of storms
so your soul won't get lost, tattered or torn.
Come kindle my soul with sweet tears of yesteryears.
For if my life is to be complete I need you,
and you can't do without me!
Can't you feel the heat?

If only for a fleeting dance
I find myself lost within the depths of your being
For who are we
but shooting stars falling from a deep blue sky!
Two solitary souls seeking shelter from
the harsh storms of this sphere.
That toss and turn like sleepy old men lost at sea.
Grant me a section of your soul
and we shall climb the highest mountain
scale the deepest sea.
That small spark within you
shall shine like the morning sun!
Refurbishing oblivious smoke into a blazing inferno
glistens brightly through the darkness.
Ignite into a sprit of God
to only follow a dream into reality!

Patricia A. Schauder

"A Ship of Dreams"

Beyond this collection box
of antique vessels of years gone by.
Priceless gems that made reality tick
once upon a time..
Is there a perfect right?
Will there ever be a total wrong?
Passing their waking minutes praying
that it won't be long until St. Peter salutes them
at that golden door!

Beyond the reflections I view in the mirror
dances dreams that might come true someday
if merely I ignore the mockery of this norm.
Visions that are docked at the side of my soul
awaiting the restless sea of realities ways.
Bless me, my Lord,
for countless are the memories of sailing ships which docked
for a time or two at the door of my soul.
Did I learn enough from each vessel I loved?
Did I care enough of the ships at sea,
drifting aimlessly around?
Is there a perfect right?
Will there ever be a total wrong?

"His Shadow"

His shadow greets me
like the morning sun.
His arms embrace me
when the day is done.
Is it a mere desire that all women have
or is it a small spark that can turn into a blazing fire?
What happens now to the mere image
of what could be,
what should be?
Oh Dear God,
is it just a fantasy?

"The Bend"

Did you ever see the light at the end of a tunnel?
The consent reminder that there's always tomorrow.
That small spark of hope at the far end of sorrow.
Did you ever recall days when you thought you had it all
yet still asked for more?
Did you ever gaze toward the sky
to merely see a victim soar?
I am who I am
by the wondrous work of God
so come join me as I travel this sod.

Oblivion!
There's nothing to it
if a being stops sharing,
daring to need me just as I am
then why be?
Did you ever demand the sightless see?
The fearless fall!
The chance of a lifetime stumbles all over the floor!
Stop!
Dance within this nightmare of obsessions
to only visualize the rainbow's end.
The silent signal that every soul must bend!

"Another Saturday night"

Seek out your visions venturing to find
that what you planned
is never entirely left behind.
If we are mere grains of sand
in the hour glass of time
allow me whisper your name
until God enchants my soul to more!
Is it merely desire that tears all souls
enabling a seed to bloom into reality's ways?
To dance and sing in the hollow halls of my mind!
Take me!
Feel me completely as I am!
For my yesteryears are gone
and tomorrows shall never come
near enough to end this illusion of mine.
Allow my intermost feelings to love you
in the depths of my dreams of you and me in mere ecstasy.

Taste a love so define until the sun refuses to shine
on a brand new morn!
And I lay awake at night
playing solitaire in my mind
wondering why?

"The Maddening Moonbeam"

And the moonbeam still shines soothing the outraged rose.
as she wept for yet another lost love.
Life goes on its merry way even if a small boy died today
or a lady of the night stopped to pray.
Why?
Why try to shine that endless spark glistening within my soul.
A black man saw it during a moment of madness
as the moon sailed passed two starry eyed silhouettes.
Can anyone caress an abnormal rose?
Do they ever climb out
from volume upon volume of forgotten lorn,
to notice a bleeding heart all tatter and torn.
The price of fame is great at times!

Did the blood come too quick for her to fully realize
that a second bud bloomed into being?
For they can't understand
the frail wonders of God's gift to man.
The beauty of a setting sun!
The enchantress of a full-grown moon!
The usefulness of a knife with a spoon!
And the moonbeam paves the way
for young love to blossom into today.

Do they ever feel the tears,
of a solitary rose such as me?
Is this merely destiny or simply a matter of fact?
Listen to a rose just before racing out the door
merely to post their fantasies,
"Must never be late!"

A moth will turn into a butterfly one day!

Give me more time and I shall pay.

A rose is a rose,

is a perfection beyond belief!

Two lovers possess that,

which is blind to the naked eye,

yet felt with each beat of their heart.

I merely sit each night and pray,

"Oh dear Lord,

will I ever fall in love?

And the moonbeam still shines,

down from the heavens above.

"A Mere Mirage"

Do we love in order to fulfill a need
that each soul strives for merely to be whole,
or do we crave that sexual act because everyone else is doing it?
Touch me tenderly in this night
as passion flares into an internal blaze
and the night was made for lovers in love.
Hold me delicately as a fine cut glass
as the flames of your lips entice that very part of me
which only desires intimacy.
Feed me!
Dress me in the silk of your smile!
Enfold my heart with the richness of your soul!
Swallow my kisses like peaceful waves
upon the ocean of life.
And the flames of forever remain but a brief moment
for the dawn woke my dreams of you
as another sunrise enters my room.

"Hear the Silence"

Voices in my mind sing silent tunes of death,
as well as praises of delight!
Oh Lord, get me through tonight?
Where would I belong
if I have no blocks to build?
No foundation to base my tomorrows on?
No melodies to my own silent song!
Why try to break this maddening throng?
No one can ever be absolutely right
yet not everyone is totally wrong?

What is that tiny spark living deep within each heart,
that must bend and tear the other apart?
Gaze deep into His endless golden sky
simply to question the whereas and the why?
Each one merely views the path
sketched out by the Mighty One's hand
to send their soul throughout this land.

Accept the fact that in order to truly gain
we must surely lose much more
Reflect that one Friday morn someone died only to be born
Reach out for a rose
yet beware of its thorns!
Each soul searches for others to belong,
as a rose thirst for His soft tears.
A sister or brother.
A friend as well as a lover!
Touch me!
Hold me till the brake of dawn,

yet don't treat me as some sexual pawn!
For what is this world's passion
but money, sex and fame!
Today's elite treat it as some game!
Win or lose we must charter a course
fitting to our soul's need's
as if we were taming a wild blue horse.
Listen to that still sweet voice
throughout a forsaken night and you may hear the praise of remorse

"A Small Room"

Seek out your fortune merely to find
that what you treasure most in life
shall forever remain hidden in your mind.
Love may burn down deep inside
yet in order for a seed to bloom.
it must first feel the rain.
So much can happen in one small room?

If only by a simple "Hi!",
my smile could venture far below
a serene wink or a tower of clay,
Touch me with a simple sigh!
Is love so blind as to seduce soft sparks
throughout my solitary self and not grant me
a certain compassionate companion?
Then release me from this Hellish life!
In my small room I turn to you.
I touch you as I kiss your soft lips,
I am one with your being
while caressing your waiting fingertip.
And why?
Nothing's perfect if we don't give it a chance?
If the music starts to play yet nobody cares to dance!
If love was mute with silence as our only embrace
let me hold you till the coming dawn!
Feel my hands as tender drops of rain
violating each painful fear,
to merely love every fragment of this flawed vessel,
as a woman, a lover, a friend!

If we only listen with our hearts
many more mountains we shall climb.
Many more song we shall sing to the end!
Many more brick walls shall slowly bend!
If only our souls could dance
to the glorious glory of natures song.
Many shall find that they truly belong!

That infernal ship which sails
across every starry eyed lover
who views that which practical minds ignore!
Hunger for that magical love sightless to the naked eye
yet known to them that truly believe!
Seek out your fortune merely to find
if you can't risk it all
it shall forever remain in your mind!

"Such is His Will"

Such is the Will of God to be born,
yes awake!
To dig graves as He takes!
The stages of life tear as well as bend
a sensitive soul such as I.
There's so much more shall meet my eye,
before greeting my Lord in the sky!

Such is the Will of God to be a part of another's heart.
To search high and low for someone to forever be there,
and know that they truly do care!
To kiss and touch the tender passions
that only God could create!

Such is the Will of God to give birth to new life,
and watch their world bloom.
To gain a knowledge blind to the naked eye
that shall be with you till the day you die!

Dear Lord please forgive this lump in my voice
for such is Your Will
as one stage slowly fades
the next evolves a bright new trill!

Patricia A. Schauder

"Between Right and Wrong"

If only by a simple gaze,
my smile could venture far beneath,
a serene wink or a tower of clay,
would you be here with me to stay?
Allow silence to be our only embrace,
as I hold you till the coming dawn!
Is there an absolute right?
Could there be a total wrong?
Let me awake by the light of tomorrow's day,
to merely feel your hands as tender drops of dew,
cherishing each fragment of this flawed being,
as a woman, a lover, a friend!
I touch you as I kiss your soft lips,
while caressing your waiting fingertip.
Nothing's perfect if we don't give it a chance?
If the music starts to play yet nobody cares to dance!
Seek out your fortune only to find,
if you can't risk it all,
it shall forever remain in your mind!

"Between Heaven and Hell"

Between Heaven and Hell,
there's a place where lovers love,
and a rose blooms at its own pace!
Soul's open their hearts without fear of disgrace!
Between each Julieent of an endless day,
thoughts of you embrace my very being.
Touch me with your gentle song,
to merely divulge that even I do belong!
Allow each facet of my being to exist,
not merely be an reflection of my soul's desire,
and notice how burning passions flare even higher!
Why must we fear the things we most desire,

Between Heaven and Hell,
there's a consent risk of giving your heart,
while others try so hard to tear it apart!
Within the core of your soul,
you held me ever so near as if we were one,
Why?
Might we live within fantasies?

Visions of your arms engulfing my solitary soul,
with the warmth of your soul,
the passion of your love?
The innocence of laughter!
The stabbing tears of goodbye!
Was it only the simple act,
two soul's play on a long, lonely night?
Oh my friend shield me from this bitter fright,
of cheerily anticipating the delicate touch,

of your arms embracing this frail rose
I am but a battered woman holding you with my mind?
Seek out your fortune merely to find,
there is a space where mourners dance,
and you'll be mine until the end of time!

"I'll be There"

Why?
Ask me again in ten thousand years,
and I shall answer once more, It's not a game!
It's a tear in the darkest of night!
It's a child consumed by fight!
Is money, fortune and fame,
all that this norm longs for?
Surely you have to lose in order to gain!
And after the shock,
the rupture of the skies,
Everyone that's born surely might die!
Can you view the wind.
as Winter appears with a bitter cry!

Stop!
No mere mortal man
will ever answer the question why?
The sun goes down while the moon stands still,
and yet I ponder, "Is it all God's Will?"
When I 'm down and feeling blue,
I simply close my eyes and think of you.
At times we crave for a hug or a smile!
Still there're moments we must be alone for awhile!
After the flames of a vision cease to be
look towards the sky and reflect on me!
Never allow this norm to sweep dreams away,
laughing hysterically as if to say,
"There's no need for foolish visions,
of caring and sharing!
Of knowing when you'll gaze back,
I'll forever be around.

Patricia A. Schauder

"A Certain Glance"

Upon a time so long ago,
I prayed to God someday we'd meet?
For deep within a tear stained night,
I sang to God the need to be whole.
The desire to expose all my life's fantasies,
into the warmth of a lover so true.
Combining the sorrow of yesterdays sadness,
with your hope for tomorrow
Take me as I truly am,
for I may never change from black to white,
or red to green and back again
Reach out for a rose yet beware of its thorns.
Seek out that magical love.
That sightless sensation binding two souls,
into one beautiful friendship achieved by a "Hi"

Upon a moment a mere glance my way,
your smile took my soul away.
Seek out your fortune and you will find,
that what you value most in life shall forever,
roam the halls of your mind.
Did you ever pray to God that your song shall soon be sung,
before laying down your soul?
Why must we meet to become a part,
only to sacrifice a portion of our heart?
Too many people treat love as if a game!
Striving for immorality, riches and fame!
One must give as well as take!
How can you hold someone when your arms shiver and shake?
Take my hand and together we shall view,

a corner of the moon as this day departs.
I glanced your way as you stolid my heart.
For upon a certain space of time,
a dream came true as I met you!

"Mardi Gras"

I rolled into a Mardi gra one Spring-like day. Many of my friends were there. "Larry, hey, you had to jump! Didn't you? I was young and you, just a year older. Why so young?" I gazed at the sky and pondered this mysterious concept called life? "Why Father, would he know me today if you hadn't needed him then!" I placed a yellow rose within his shadow and strolled on.

"Grandma," I yelled! "Grandma, you know you made the best home-made noodles I ever tasted? Remember when your son married my mom? You never forgave her for that! You were forever calling me Patsy to get back at mom for taking your only child away! You answered your phone once too many times! That last call was a killer! They didn't even let me see you sleep! Claimed I was too young?" I looked toward the sun. "Did she ever really know me?"

"Grandpa," I hurried towards him. "I never knew how to talk to you yet I know you were the greatest key-smith in town! True, maybe you were the only key-smith but you were the best!" I gave a white rose to him. "You know, everyone in our house woke up five minutes before they called about you. Dad cried! Second time in my life that I saw Dad cry. He loved you! Did he ever tell you that? Most men don't show emotion! Pity, even Christ wept! Are they too proud? Too manly to reveal to others that they, also, need a hug at times?" I glanced beyond the picket fence to glimpse at a lover waiting to take me far into the future. "Can I really give him what he wants? I want to yet I never did before!"

I strolled around Ralph, a small but mighty guy. "Your mouth was the biggest part on you. If I would have never went home for Christmas, would you still be here today? Your parents neglected to love you but I didn't!" I laid a soft rose beside him. "They found mice in your hair and you were skin and bones when they placed you at that home. I recall you told those who came to care for you that you were supposed to be dead! How morbid! Going through life telling people that you shouldn't be here. And every year you would watch that tel-a-thon all night long. Jerry's kids! Ha! All that money and you still ended up here! And on Christmas morning too! Did you finally play baseball? Did God eventually grant you that wish you had about a woman on your lap?" I rolled slowly past. There were deep black clouds over head.

"And sometimes when we touch, the honesty's too much." I softly sang. "Jim, I thought we never would meet again! You wanted to marry me! We would be the first to go to meals and the last to leave! We could talk about anything and get lost in any subject. I miss that!" And then I glanced only to find him staring straight at me, as if to say, "Forget the past with all those lost affairs! They loved you then but I want you now!"

Drops escaped the innermost walls of my mind as I rolled on towards a face without a bottle. "Dad," I screamed as I reached out my spastic arms. "you're finally sober! There's so much I need to tell you! I'm moving to Toledo this fall. Yes, Dad, I'm moving closer to Julie. I still wonder what your reaction would be? The whole family seems to be slightly concern about my upcoming living situation? I think they are like much of society? Did you ever understand my physical disability? I wonder? If I came out "normal", would relationships be different? We never really talked! I just watched the grass grow with you and saw you drink your life away!" My face was wet with tears as I laid a glass rose at his side. "I wish you had hugged me more? Did you hear I'm published again? This makes the 15th time." The rain began to pour as I stared at the black sky. "Lord, did I give him enough love?" I slowly rolled around a tall oak tree. The wind started to blow with anger.

"Jerry," I stopped my chair. "I was just getting to feel good talking to you when I woke up one night to hear all these voices discussing your departure. Some were strange, talking as if you were merely a number! You were as human as I am! I remember how red your ears got whenever your temper flared. There was also familiar voices that didn't know exactly what to say?" I looked up. The lover's eyes embraced me as if he was comforting me in some way. "Does anyone actually know how another feels? They can merely guess! I dropped a pink rose at his side. "You really knew the Bible. I admired you for that! We never fully know what we have until we lose it." A ray of light broke through the clouds. Drops were still dancing on my face. "Where's the rainbow, God? Your Word said you'll give me what I want so why am I unfastening all my close knit ties?" I looked at the gate. His eyes were calling me.

The wind turned into a gentle breeze as I reached the gate. The softness of his eyes reminded me that the past only holds memories of what will never be again. The future is merely dreams meant for praying to God that he can only grant. Don't lead, I may not follow! Don't follow, I may not lead! Just roll beside me and give me your today!

About the Author

Shake, Rattle & a Cinnamon Roll is about a woman born with severe Cerebral Palsy, told in fictional form. She was born when people really didn't understand Cerebral Palsy and wanted to put her in an institution. Thanks to her parents that didn't happen. She also wrote Shake, Rattle and a Cinnamon Roll to inform people that, in spite of her limitations, she still leads a very productive life. She was born in Toledo, Ohio; raised in Battle Creek, Michigan; and spent time in Warsaw, Ohio; yet now reside back in Toledo.

Someone asked her once, "How would you sell yourself?" In reply, she simply replied, "Take a look, and see what you will miss, if you don't read my book." She is certainly not rich, well educated or famous. This is my story and these are my verses. Take it or leave it. The choice is yours.

Printed in the United States
41236LVS00006B/1-39